Diabetes Management

Diabetes Management

A MANUAL FOR PATIENT-CENTRED CARE

Janet Titchener

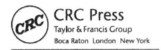

CRC Press
Taylor & Francis Group
Boca Raton London New York

CRC Press is an imprint of the
Taylor & Francis Group, an **informa** business

First edition published 2020
by CRC Press
6000 Broken Sound Parkway NW, Suite 300, Boca Raton, FL 33487-2742

and by CRC Press
2 Park Square, Milton Park, Abingdon, Oxon, OX14 4RN

Library of Congress Cataloging-in-Publication Data
Names: Titchener, Janet, 1957– author.
Title: Diabetes management: a manual for patient-centred care / by Janet Titchener.
Description: First edition. | Boca Raton: CRC Press, 2020. |
Includes bibliographical references and index. |
Summary: "Diabetes is a chronic disease involving self-management by the patients.
This book teaches providers the skills to translate and transfer complex medical information to empower
patients to participate in making well informed decisions about their own care on a daily basis,
as directed by the American Diabetes Association" – Provided by publisher.
Identifiers: LCCN 2020002773 (print) | LCCN 2020002774 (ebook) |
ISBN 9780367344931 (pbk) | ISBN 9780367897628 (hbk) | ISBN 9780429326196 (ebk)
Subjects: MESH: Diabetes Mellitus–therapy | Self Care | Patient-Centered Care |
Self Management | Patient Education as Topic
Classification: LCC RC660.4 (print) | LCC RC660.4 (ebook) |
NLM WK 815 | DDC 616.4/6206–dc23
LC record available at https://lccn.loc.gov/2020002773
LC ebook record available at https://lccn.loc.gov/2020002774

ISBN: 978-0-367-89762-8 (hbk)
ISBN: 978-0-367-34493-1 (pbk)
ISBN: 978-0-429-32619-6 (ebk)

Dedication

This book is dedicated to all those with diabetes who shared their stories with me as well as their experience of what it means to live with diabetes. Without your sharing, I would never have gained the insight and understanding so critical to providing a patient-centred approach to diabetes care.

Janet Titchener

Dedication

Contents

Patient handouts

About the author

Janet Titchener, MD, is a graduate of Otago University (Diploma, Physical Education), University of Connecticut (Masters, Psychology), Thomas Jefferson University (Masters, Physiotherapy) and The University of Pennsylvania School of Medicine (Doctorate of Medicine).

Convinced that successful medical care could only be achieved if diseases were managed within the context of the patient, Dr Titchener chose to train as a Family Practice Physician (Lancaster General, University of Pennsylvania). During her residency and fellowship she subspecialised in diabetology and is currently Board Certified in Advanced Diabetes Management through the American Association of Diabetes Educators.

As Medical Director of GPSI Diabetes Ltd, Dr Titchener provides care for all types of diabetes, across all age groups. Her clinical practice adheres to the principles of patient-centred clinical medicine so that each patient is considered the expert with regard to knowing which management approach will best fit with their life and life's choices.

Dr Titchener is the recipient of the 2010 Eli Lilly/NZSSD Primary–Secondary Physician award for her clinical work and teaching within GPSI Diabetes Ltd, New Zealand.

Introduction

"Diabetes is, in many ways, a large part of the future of medicine"

Fowler MJ *Clinical Diabetes* 2010:28:42–46

Diabetes has become a major international public health problem.[1] The number of people with diabetes is estimated to be 425 million and is predicted to increase to 629 million by 2045.[2] As increasing incidence and prevalence overburdens healthcare systems, it is arguably the most significant challenge in healthcare today.[3] Limitations in workforce, resources and funding are the reasons most often given for poor management.[4,5] However, more recently, the current conventional model of healthcare itself has been recognised as a significant barrier to good diabetes care.[6,7] Having evolved to manage acute episodic illness, it is ill suited to approaching the complexities of a chronic disease.

Chronic disease is more complex than acute disease, both medically and psychosocially. Chronic diseases are multiple-organ diseases requiring skills for preventative as well as current disease management; these are lifelong diseases where emphasis is on control not cure, requiring monitoring with constant attention to medication management; these are illnesses which a person has to live with and independently manage on a daily basis, meaning that key treatment decisions (e.g. lifestyle change, taking medication regularly) are entirely under their control; and finally, as each person is a unique autonomous individual with their own set of beliefs and priorities about their life, these are illnesses where management success does not occur if the treatments being selected do not suit the patient's unique life-situations and cultural and personal beliefs.[8–10]

Recognising the influence psychosocial factors have on disease management, and stimulated by studies demonstrating the effectiveness of patient self-management, new models of care are shifting from treatment that is done to passive recipients by medical experts, to patient-centred care where management decisions result from a collaborative partnership between provider and patient with the patient actively participating in disease management choices.[11] Indeed, since 2012, recommendations for diabetes management from both the American Diabetes Association and the European Association for the Study of Diabetes have stopped advocating one management option over another. Rather, they ask that management choices "be considered within the context of the needs, preferences, and tolerances of each patient", emphasising that "individualization of treatment is the cornerstone of success".[12]

To provide patient-centred diabetes care a provider needs to develop two skills: first, a good understanding of the pathophysiology of diabetes, the differences and similarities between the different types of diabetes, and an excellent understanding of how the medications and insulins target different pathophysiologies and work synergistically to control blood sugars; and second, the skills to transfer this same knowledge to patients, enabling the patient to participate in management decisions and empowering them to self-manage their disease. This manual sets out to teach providers both sets of skills.

The first half of the manual provides basic knowledge around the pathophysiology of diabetes and different management options. The second half then presents information on how foods affect blood sugars and how to address cardiovascular risk factors. The information is presented in such a way as to assist the reader in developing their skills for translating complex medical knowledge into understandable lay language during a patient-centred consultation. Techniques are also provided to enhance a provider's patient-centred skills for the transfer of knowledge to the patient and for successful engagement in a partnership of care.

REFERENCES

1. Boyle JP, Honeycutt AA, Narayan KM, et al. Projection of diabetes burden through 2050: impact of changing demographic and disease prevalence in the US. Diabetes Care. 2001;24:1936–1940
2. International Diabetes Federation. IDF Diabetes Atlas, 8th ed (internet), 2017. Available on www.diabetesatlas.org. Accessed 17 May 2019
3. Singh D. Transforming chronic care: evidence about improving care for people with long term conditions. Health Services Management Centre, University of Birmingham, 2006
4. Selby JV, Ray GT, Zhang D, Colby CJ. Excess costs of medical care for patients with diabetes in a managed care population. Diabetes Care. 1997;20:1396–1402
5. Shahady E. The Florida Diabetes Master Clinician Program: facilitating increased quality and significant cost savings for diabetic patients. Clin Diabetes. 2008;26:29–33
6. Janes R, Titchener J, Pere J, et al. Understanding barriers to glycaemic control from the patient's perspective. J Prim Health Care. 2013;5:114–122
7. Kahn R, Anderson JE. Improving diabetes care: the model of health care reform. Diabetes Care. 2009;32:1115–1118
8. Laffel LM, Vangsness L, Connell A, et al. Impact of ambulatory, family-focused teamwork intervention on glycemic control in youth with type 1 diabetes. J Pediatrics. 2003;142:409–416
9. Rother ML, O'Connor AM. Health decisions and decision support for women. Annu Rev Public Health. 2003;24:413–433
10. Simpson EL, House AO. Involving users in the delivery and evaluation of mental health services: a systematic review. BMJ. 2002;325:1265–1268
11. Glasgow RE, Peeples M, Skovlund SE. Where is the patient in diabetes performance measures? The case for including patient-centered and self-management measures. Diabetes Care. 2008;31:1046–1050
12. Inzucchi SE, Bergenstal RM, Buse JB, et al. Management of hyperglycemia in type 2 diabetes: a patient-centred approach. Position statement of the American Diabetes Association (ADA) and the European Association for the Study of Diabetes (EASD). Diabetes Care. 2012;35:1364–1379

The physiology of glucose metabolism

The body is made up of millions of cells. Each cell can be thought of as an engine with a specific job to do – brain cells think, kidney cells make urine, cells in the eye are for seeing, and so on. Like any engine, these cells require fuel to run on. The main fuel that the cells in our body run on is glucose (a simple sugar).

Glucose is transported within the blood and delivered to the cells via blood vessels. The glucose enters each cell through glucose-specific channels or "gates". For most cells in the body, cellular uptake of glucose can only occur in the presence of insulin, as insulin is needed for opening the gates. In muscle cells, glucose-specific channels can also be opened by exercise (Figure 1.1). Brain cells are the only cells that can receive glucose without assistance from insulin or any other mechanism.

THERE ARE TWO SOURCES OF GLUCOSE

Our body has two major sources of glucose:

- a continual supply from the liver, and
- a sporadic supply from intestinal absorption of ingested food.

To ensure that there is always a constant supply of glucose available for cells, the body has several places where glucose can be stored and/or generated. The largest and most important of these is the liver. The liver stores glycogen (a storage form of glucose). During fasting, glycogen is broken down into glucose and released into the blood – a process called glycogenolysis. The liver is also capable of making glucose, a process called gluconeogenesis. Through glycogenolysis and gluconeogenesis, the liver constantly releases glucose into the blood, ensuring that fuel is available for the body's cells 24 hours a day (Figure 1.2).

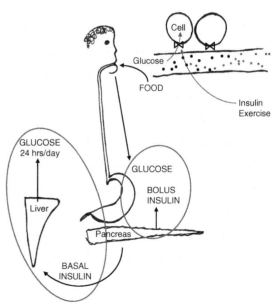

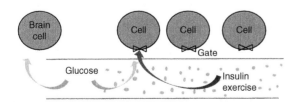

Figure 1.1 Glucose enters cells through a glucose-specific 'gate', but can only do so if insulin or exercise is also present.

Figure 1.2 Two sources of glucose (hepatic and ingestion of foods) are matched by a basal and bolus secretion of insulin from the pancreas.

The second source of glucose is from food. When food is digested, it is broken down into the basic metabolic components of carbohydrates, proteins and fats. These are either used immediately or stored as energy for future use. Ingested carbohydrates (along with a small percentage of ingested protein) are directly converted into glucose in the gut and absorbed into the blood. This blood glucose is taken up immediately by the body's cells to support bodily functions (e.g. walking, thinking, pumping of the heart), cellular repair and growth. Some of the glucose is transported to the liver to replenish stores and, if we eat more than is needed for current cellular function, the glucose is converted into long-term energy stores – i.e. the person gains weight.

THERE ARE TWO 'KINDS' OF INSULIN – BASAL AND BOLUS

As noted above, except in the brain and in exercising muscle, cellular uptake of glucose can only occur in the presence of insulin. Insulin is a hormone secreted from the pancreatic β-cells. When released into the blood, the insulin binds to specific receptors on the surface of the cells causing the glucose-specific 'gate' on the cell membrane wall to open so glucose can enter the cell (Figure 1.2).

Just as glucose is supplied in two different ways, the pancreas provides insulin in two different ways. To match the constant glucose secretion from the liver, the pancreas produces a constant 'drip' of insulin, known as the basal insulin (Figure 1.2). The production of pancreatic basal insulin and hepatic glucose are beautifully matched with each other by hormonal feedback loop systems (counter-regulatory systems). This ensures that there is no under- or oversupply of glucose from the liver, and that any glucose released from the liver is appropriately taken up by the cells. Thus, in a person who does not have diabetes, blood sugar levels remain within a narrow range – between 3.5 and 7.8 mmol/L (65–140 mg/dL).

In response to the rapid influx of glucose following a meal, the pancreas immediately releases 'pre-packaged' insulin – referred to as a bolus of insulin (Figure 1.2). Depending on the content of the meal, this is then followed by increased insulin synthesis and release, again carefully regulated to match circulating glucose concentrations. This prompt pancreatic action ensures that the cellular glucose uptake can occur instantly and efficiently,

which is why the postprandial blood glucose of a person without diabetes does not rise above 7.8 mmol/L (140 mg/dL) regardless of meal volume or content.

OTHER HORMONES ASSIST WITH GLUCOSE HOMEOSTASIS

As our understanding of glucose metabolism has grown, we now know that this representation of insulin as the sole regulator of glucose metabolism is too simplistic. Glucose homeostasis (i.e. keeping blood glucose within normal range) involves multiple pancreatic (insulin, glucagon, amylin) and incretin (gut) hormones (GIP, GLP-1; see below), and there may well be more yet to be discovered (Figure 1.3).

Glucagon This hormone is secreted from the pancreatic α-cells which sit next to the insulin-producing β-cells. Glucagon's major role is to stimulate hepatic glucose production during the fasting state or when blood sugars go low. During and immediately following a meal, glucagon secretion is suppressed to ensure hepatic glucose output is reduced, as the body does not need two simultaneous sources of glucose.

Amylin This is another pancreatic hormone. It is co-secreted with insulin from the pancreatic

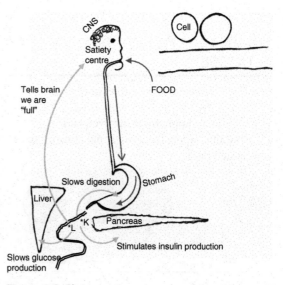

Figure 1.3 The incretin system has four targets – the central nervous system (CNS), the stomach, the pancreas and the liver.

β-cells following the ingestion of food. Amylin suppresses postprandial glucagon secretion, thereby decreasing glucagon-stimulated hepatic glucose output (as described above). Amylin also slows the rate of gastric emptying. This reduces the rate at which glucose is delivered to the small intestine for absorption, thereby playing an important role in the control of postprandial blood sugars. By slowing gastric emptying, it is also possible that amylin reduces food intake and body weight – i.e. amylin has similar actions to the incretin hormones (see below).

Incretin (gut) hormones Simplistically, the incretin system can be viewed as an overall coordinator of glucose homeostasis following a meal. Several incretin hormones have now been characterised. The two most significant are GIP (gastric inhibitory polypeptide) and GLP-1 (glucagon-like peptide 1), with GLP-1 considered more physiologically relevant in humans. Both are secreted from cells in the gut (the 'K' and 'L' cells) following the ingestion of food. The K cells are primarily located in the proximal part of the small intestine (duodenum and jejunum), while the L cells are located more distally in the ileum.

The incretin hormones have four actions (Figure 1.3). They

- Stimulate insulin secretion from the pancreatic β-cells (to match incoming food).
- Inhibit glucagon secretion from the pancreatic α-cells (thereby reducing hepatic glucose production).
- Slow gastric emptying (thereby reducing postprandial glucose excursion).
- Stimulate the satiety centre in the central nervous system, i.e. help control appetite.

THE KIDNEYS ALSO PLAY A CRUCIAL ROLE

The kidneys, like the liver, have glucose stores and contribute to the supply of glucose during periods of fasting. However, the kidneys' main contribution to glucose homeostasis is through their ability to reabsorb blood glucose that has been filtered through the glomeruli.

The kidneys act as the body's filter system (Figure 1.4), playing an important role in maintaining the constitution of our blood. Each time the blood circulates around the body, it passes through the glomeruli within the kidneys. The glomeruli act like a filter: large proteins in the blood (e.g. red blood cells, platelets, immunoglobulins) do not pass through the filter and remain in the blood vessel, while the smaller components (e.g. electrolytes, water, glucose) do pass through the filter and into the renal tubules. The tubules are then responsible for determining whether these

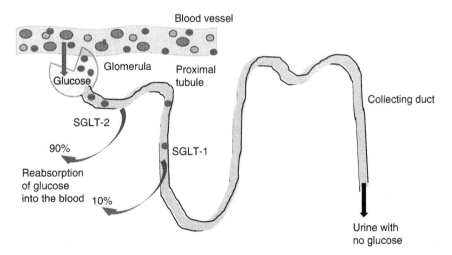

Figure 1.4 Blood is filtered by the kidneys. In the glomeruli, glucose passes from the blood into renal tubules. The sodium-dependent glucose transporter (SGLT) transports the glucose back into the bloodstream.

smaller components should be transported back into the blood or whether they should be excreted.

In a healthy kidney, 100% of the glucose in the blood passes through the glomeruli and into the tubules. But, as glucose is our fuel, the tubules transport 100% of the glucose back into the blood and no sugar appears in the urine. The transporting is done by the sodium-dependent glucose transporter (SGLT) cells located in the proximal renal tubules. Of note, there is a threshold to how much glucose the SGLT cells can transport, so that if they are presented with too much glucose – such as in a person with poorly controlled diabetes – not all the glucose will be transported back to the blood and the surplus continues down the tubules and appears in the person's urine (glucosuria).

SUMMARY

- The cells in our body require a fuel; this fuel is glucose.
- There are two main sources of glucose: a constant 24-hour supply from the liver and a sporadic influx from the ingestion of food.

- Cellular uptake of glucose requires insulin. This is supplied by the pancreas in two different ways: as basal insulin, a 24-hour 'drip' to match hepatic glucose output; and as bolus insulin, delivered at mealtimes to match the sporadic glucose influx from food digestion.
- Maintaining glucose homeostasis is complex and involves the liver, the kidneys and the interplay of multiple pancreatic and gut hormones.

REFERENCES

1. Aronoff SL, Berkowitz K, Shreiner B, Want L. Glucose metabolism and regulation: beyond insulin and glucagon. Diabetes Spectr. 2004; 17:183–190
2. Fonseca VA. Clinical diabetes: translating research into practice. Saunders Elsevier, Philadelphia, 2006
3. Chao EC. SGLT-2 Inhibitors: a new mechanism for glycemic control. Clin Diabetes. 2014;32:4–11

2

The pathophysiology of diabetes

Until relatively recently, diabetes was defined as "a group of metabolic diseases characterised by hyperglycemia resulting from defects in insulin secretion, insulin action, or both."[1] However, our understanding of the pathophysiology of diabetes continues to evolve, and it is now recognised that multiple pathologies, not just defects in insulin secretion and action, contribute to the development of hyperglycaemia.

As outlined in the previous chapter, glucose metabolism is highly complex: it involves multiple organs and multiple endocrine systems. Such complexity provides considerable opportunity for something to go wrong: a pancreas may cease to produce insulin because of an autoimmune destruction of β-cells (e.g. type 1 diabetes), or because of a deposition disease (e.g. haemochromatosis), or because of trauma. Reduced insulin supplies could also be due to reduced insulin production secondary to a missing component in the insulin manufacturing process (e.g. monogenic diabetes). Perhaps there is nothing wrong with pancreatic insulin production, and an apparent insulin 'deficiency' is the result of insulin resistance due to cellular receptors not responding appropriately to available insulin. It is important to understand that at diagnosis, a person may have one disruption or pathology in the metabolic pathway or may have multiple pathologies.

Another important understanding is that the combination of pathologies contributing to hyperglycaemia at diagnosis may change over time. For example, at diagnosis a person with type 1 diabetes will have low insulin production due to autoimmune destruction of the β-cells, but over the years may develop insulin resistance due to weight gain; while early on in the evolution of type 2 diabetes a person may have excessive insulin production to overcome peripheral insulin resistance, but later become insulin-deficient secondary to a progressively failing pancreas. So, the type of diabetes a person has does not accurately define their underlying pathology; and two people with the same type of diabetes may have very different underlying pathologies.

Similarly, while the underlying aetiology of two types of diabetes can be entirely different, the resulting pathologies could be identical. As outlined above, a person with insulin deficiency due to an autoimmune destruction of pancreatic β-cells (type 1 diabetes) may become obese and develop insulin resistance, while a person with type 2 diabetes and insulin resistance may well progress to having significant pancreatic deficiency. Clearly, because of this 'sharing' of pathologies, the same management options are being used for completely different types of diabetes.

As hyperglycaemia is the result of many different pathological mechanisms, the disease of diabetes is really a large, heterogeneous group of diseases and classifying them has been difficult and, at times, controversial.[2] The American Diabetes Association catagorises the different known types according to the underlying cause or aetiology of hyperglycaemia, listing four general categories of diabetes:[3]

- Type 1 diabetes – an autoimmune destruction of β-cells resulting in insulin deficiency.
- Type 2 diabetes – hyperglycaemia due to multiple underlying pathologies but usually described as progressive loss of β-cell function against a background of insulin resistance. It may range from predominant insulin resistance with relative insulin deficiency to a predominant insulin secretory defect with some insulin resistance.

- Types of diabetes due to rare and not so rare causes, including genetic defects of the β-cell, genetic defects of insulin action, diseases of the exocrine pancreas, endocrinopathies and drug-or chemical-induced diabetes.
- Gestational diabetes – diabetes diagnosed in the second or third trimester of pregnancy.

In a primary care setting most patients with diabetes fall into one of the first two categories. However, having a basic understanding of other types of diabetes is important to minimise the risk of missing an alternative diagnosis that could significantly change management decisions and ultimately improve clinical outcomes.

TYPE 1 DIABETES

Type 1 diabetes is the result of an autoimmune process that targets the pancreatic β-cells that produce insulin. Type 1 diabetes accounts for 5–10% of all those with diabetes, although this can be much higher in some ethnic groups (e.g. in the Scandinavian countries).[3] The incidence of type 1 diabetes is increasing.[1]

As with other autoimmune diseases, people with type 1 diabetes are born with a genetic predisposition to getting the disease. It is believed that a superimposed environmental trigger initiates the autoimmune process. While a strong association has been demonstrated between individuals who develop type 1 diabetes and specific sets of genetic markers, there is no clear understanding of what the environmental trigger might be. Various triggers have been suggested (e.g. viruses, food additives, cow's milk), but none of them has been proven to have a clear cause-and-effect association with the development of type 1 diabetes.

Importantly, having the genetic markers does not guarantee the development of diabetes. Furthermore, 80–90% of all new diagnoses occur in individuals with no family history of type 1 diabetes, although other family members may have other autoimmune disorders and people with type 1 diabetes are susceptible to developing other autoimmune disorders.[1] If there is a family history of type 1 diabetes, there is a 15- to 20-fold increased risk of a first-degree relative subsequently developing type 1 diabetes.[4]

Historically, type 1 diabetes was considered a childhood disease. However, autoimmune diabetes can develop at any age, even in the eighth and ninth decades. Indeed, over half of the people with type 1 diabetes are over the age of 30 at diagnosis.[1] Various terms such as 'latent autoimmune diabetes of the adult' (LADA), 'latent type 1 diabetes', 'slowly progressive insulin-dependent diabetes', 'type 1.5 diabetes' and 'antibody-positive phenotypic type 2 diabetes' have been used in the past to describe adult-onset diabetes with positive antibodies.[5] However, because it is now recognised that autoimmune destruction of β-cells can occur at any age, classifying adult-onset autoimmune diabetes as a separate entity from conventional type 1 diabetes has been challenged and is no longer considered appropriate.[3,5]

The autoimmune destruction of β-cells leads to a progressive decline in pancreatic insulin secretion. The rate of β-cell decline ('honeymoon period') can vary considerably between individuals, as can the completeness of β-cell destruction: i.e. following the honeymoon period, some patients may have more residual β-cell function than others.[3,5] Only when 80% of the β-cells have been destroyed do patients develop the first clinical symptoms of diabetes. These include thirst, urinary frequency and urinary ketones with or without ketoacidosis.

As type 1 diabetes can occur at any age, and with the increasing incidence of children developing type 2 diabetes, the age of the patient alone can no longer be used as verification of the type of diabetes. Furthermore, with a worldwide obesity epidemic, body habitus has become a very poor indicator of the type of diabetes. A child or adult can be obese and develop autoimmune diabetes. This makes distinguishing between type 1 and type 2 diabetes challenging, and confirmation of type 1 diabetes should be made by checking antibodies at the time of diagnosis (see Chapter 3, Making the Diagnosis of Diabetes).

While the presence of antibodies confirms type 1 diabetes, up to 20% of people currently labelled as having type 1 do not have measurable antibodies at diagnosis. Of course, it is possible that these people have a different aetiology to their diabetes. Indeed, reports suggest that up to 5% of youth carrying the diagnosis of type 1 diabetes actually have monogenic diabetes (see below).[6]

TYPE 2 DIABETES

Until relatively recently, the primary pathology underlying type 2 diabetes was thought to be peripheral insulin resistance reducing a cell's ability to take up glucose. Initially, to overcome this insulin resistance and keep blood sugars within normal range, pancreatic β-cells increase insulin production. Over time, however, β-cells begin to fail and the reduced insulin levels are no longer sufficient to overcome cellular insulin resistance; the cells are no longer able to take up glucose, blood sugar levels rise and the person is diagnosed with diabetes. Thus, historically, type 2 diabetes was thought to present as hyperinsulinemia (pancreatic sufficiency) with relative insulin deficiency secondary to insulin resistance, later progressing to pancreatic insufficiency with absolute insulin deficiency.

However, as more is understood about type 2 diabetes, we now realise that an essential component for the development of type 2 diabetes is impaired β-cell function – not just insulin resistance.[3,7] In fact, at the time of diagnosis, individuals with type 2 diabetes already have a 60% reduction in β-cell mass, while those diagnosed with glucose intolerance have a 40% reduction in β-cell mass. Of note, β-cell function continues to decline over time, and it is this decline, not worsening insulin resistance, that is primarily responsible for the progression of type 2 diabetes.[8]

The pathologies contributing to β-cell decline in type 2 diabetes are not well understood, although, as with type 1 diabetes, both genetic and environmental factors play a role.[3,9] Numerous genetic markers for type 2 diabetes have been identified and, not surprisingly, most appear to be related to β-cell dysfunction.[10]

Obesity and lack of exercise along with other environmental factors are clearly major contributors to the development of type 2 diabetes as they increase peripheral insulin resistance and contribute to pancreatic demise. The mechanisms by which these increase insulin resistance and pancreatic dysfunction are also not well understood. However, as outlined above, it is important to understand that obesity and lack of exercise alone do not cause diabetes. Indeed, many obese, inactive people do not develop type 2 diabetes.[10] For type 2 diabetes to develop there must be an underlying pancreatic β-cell insufficiency. The determining factor as to whether a person develops type 2 diabetes is their baseline pancreatic function: if a person has excellent pancreatic function, a considerable number of poor lifestyle choices (e.g. poor diet, smoking, weight gain) will be required before enough insulin resistance develops to elevate blood sugars, whereas in a person with a relatively low-functioning pancreas, only one poor lifestyle choice may be all that is needed to create enough insulin resistance to initiate hyperglycaemia.

Aside from peripheral insulin resistance and pancreatic β-cell insufficiency, people with type 2 diabetes also lose the sophisticated counter-regulatory systems mediated by glucagon, amylin and the incretins. This results in increased hepatic glucose output and dysregulation of glucose management during ingestion of food.[11,12]

Unfortunately, unlike for type 1 diabetes, there are no specific blood tests to confirm a diagnosis of type 2 diabetes. Establishing the diagnosis is based on the clinical presentation of the patient, such as age at diagnosis, body habitus, the presence or absence of metabolic syndrome, and so on. Yet, as noted earlier, basing a diagnosis on clinical presentation is problematic, especially with the growing obesity epidemic. Until 15 or 20 years ago, type 2 diabetes accounted for less than 3% of all new cases of diabetes in children. Today, 45% of new paediatric cases in the United States and 80% of all new paediatric cases in Japan are of type 2 diabetes,[13,14] while, as noted above, new-onset diabetes during the adult years can no longer be presumed to be type 2 diabetes. In fact, it is believed that 20% of adults currently carrying the diagnosis of type 2 diabetes do not have type 2 diabetes.[15] Chapter 7 reviews the clinical expectations of the various types of diabetes to assist providers to more accurately categorise their patients.

MONOGENIC DIABETES

Monogenic diabetes encompasses a heterogeneous group of diabetes that, as the name implies, are caused by a single gene defect or chromosomal abnormality within the β-cell resulting in impaired insulin secretion.[16] Monogenic diabetes includes MODY (maturity-onset diabetes of the young), neonatal diabetes and mitochondrial diabetes. Multiple genetic mutations have now been identified resulting in many different types of monogenic diabetes. However, four types of monogenic diabetes, associated with mutations in the *HNF1A*, *HNF1B*, *HNF4A* and *GCK* genes, account for 90% of all cases.

Monogenic diabetes typically shows up prior to the age of 25, although diagnosis can often be missed and delayed by 10 years.[17] The genetic mutations can be sporadic, or inherited in a recessive or dominant manner, and should be suspected if diabetes occurs in multiple family members within two, three or more generations.[16,18]

Monogenic diabetes is believed to account for 2–5% of all cases of diabetes.[17] However, because monogenic diabetes is rarely considered as a possibility at diagnosis, currently the majority of cases are undiagnosed; some 80% are thought to be misclassified as type 1 or type 2 diabetes.[18] A negative antibody test in someone presenting like a type 1 should raise suspicion for monogenic diabetes, as should a young adult presenting with atypical type 2 diabetes (i.e. not obese, not insulin-dependent). If monogenic diabetes is suspected, genetic screening is recommended to ensure appropriate treatment.[19]

GESTATIONAL DIABETES

Diabetes diagnosed in the second or third trimester of pregnancy, with no evidence of pregestational diabetes, is classified as gestational diabetes (GDM). During mid-to-late pregnancy there is an increase in insulin resistance due to placental hormones and maternal weight gain. There is also increased clearance of insulin by the placenta. To meet the increased insulin needs, a healthy woman in her third trimester must produce 65% more insulin.[20] Thus, while several factors are thought to contribute to the development of GDM, an essential contributing component must necessarily be underlying pancreatic insufficiency.[21] Following the delivery of the baby, increased insulin needs to resolve and the woman's blood sugars return to normal. However, developing GDM is an indicator of underlying pancreatic insufficiency and a powerful predictor of diabetes later in life.

Infrequently, autoimmune (type 1) or other types of diabetes may present as new onset during pregnancy.

OTHER TYPES OF DIABETES

To date, more than 50 different types of diabetes have been recognised – most rare, but some with increasing prevalence. A review of all of these is beyond the scope of this manual. However, it is important to keep in mind that, while type 1 diabetes is our most often cited reason for pancreatic β-cell insufficiency, any disease that affects the whole pancreas will necessarily cause β-cell insufficiency. Haemochromatosis has always been the textbook example of pancreatic insufficiency due to

causes other than type 1 diabetes. However, haemochromatosis as a cause of diabetes is rare these days due to the regularity of screening blood tests, which frequently include liver function tests. Subsequent work-up of elevated liver function values will result in early diagnosis of haemochromatosis before pancreatic damage occurs.

One cause of pancreatic insufficiency that is contributing to the increasing incidence of diabetes is chronic pancreatitis secondary to alcohol, gallstones and/or obesity. Medications for tuberculosis, HIV/AIDs and modern biologics are also contributing to the incidence of diabetes secondary to pancreatic insufficiency.

SUMMARY

- Diabetes is a group of metabolic diseases characterised by hyperglycaemia secondary to one or more pathologies.
- While type 1 diabetes and type 2 diabetes are the most common types, there are many other types of diabetes – some rare and some not so rare.
- Diabetes, regardless of type, is a progressive disease and the pathologies contributing to its expression can change over time.
- Different types of diabetes do not share aetiologies but may share similar pathologies: a person with type 1 diabetes and a person with type 2 diabetes can both have insulin deficiency and insulin resistance secondary to obesity.
- Type 1 diabetes is an autoimmune disease. The person is born with a genetic predisposition to developing the disease but only develops diabetes following a superimposed environmental hit. Autoimmune diabetes can occur at any age.
- Type 2 diabetes is due to a number of heterogeneous pathologies. However, reduced β-cell mass is necessary for the development of diabetes and is also the primary contributor to disease progression. Poor lifestyle choices alone do not cause type 2 diabetes.

REFERENCES

1. American Diabetes Association. Diagnosis and classification of diabetes mellitus [position statement]. Diabetes Care. 2014;37(suppl1):s81–90
2. Gale EA. Declassifying diabetes. Diabetologia. 2006;49:1989–1995
3. American Diabetes Association. Classification and diagnosis of diabetes: standards of medical care in diabetes – 2019. Diabetes Care. 2019;42(suppl 1): s13–28
4. Fonseca VA. Clinical diabetes: translating research into practice. Saunders Elsevier, Philadelphia, 2006
5. Stenstrom G, Gottsater A, Bakhtadze E, et al. Latent autoimmune diabetes in adults. Definition, prevalence, β-cell function and treatment. Diabetes. 2005;54(suppl 2):s68–72
6. Gilliam LK, Pihoker C, Ellard S, et al. Unrecognised maturity-onset diabetes of the young (MODY) due to HNF1-alpha mutations in the SEARCH for Diabetes in Youth Study. Diabetes. 2007;56(suppl1):s74–s75
7. Kanat M, Winnier D, et al. The relationship between β-cell function and glycated haemoglobin. Results from the veterans administration genetic epidemiology study. Diabetes Care. 2011;34:1006–1010
8. DeFronzo RA, Abdul-Ghani M. Type 2 Diabetes can be prevented with early pharmacological intervention. Diabetes Care. 2011;34:s202–209
9. D'Adamo E, Caprio S. Type 2 diabetes in youth: epidemiology and pathophysiology. Diabetes Care. 2011;34:s161–s165
10. Eckel RH, Kahn SE, Ferrannini E, et al. Obesity and type 2 diabetes: what can be unified and what needs to be individualized? Diabetes Care. 2011;34:1424–1430
11. Gastaldelli A, Toschi E, Pettiti M, et al. Effect of physiological hyperinsulinemia on gluconeogenesis in nondiabetic subjects and in type 2 diabetic patients. Diabetes. 2001;50:1807–1812
12. Wahren J, Ekberg K. Splanchnic regulation of glucose production. Annu Rev Nutr. 2007;27:329–345
13. Pinhas-Hamiel O, Zeitler P. The global spread of type 2 diabetes mellitus in children and adolescents. J Pediatr. 2005;146:693–700
14. Pinhas-Hamiel O, Zeitler P. Acute and chronic complications of type 2 diabetes mellitus in children and adolescents. Lancet. 2007;369:1823–1831
15. Qi X, Sun J, et al. Prevalence and correlates of latent autoimmune diabetes in adults in Tianjin, China. Diabetes Care. 2011;34:66–70
16. Fajans SS. Scope and heterogeneous nature of MODY. Diabetes Care. 1990;13:49–64
17. Henzen C. Monogenic diabetes mellitus due to defects in insulin secretion. Swiss Med Wkly. 2012;142:w13690
18. Draznin D, Philipson LH, McGill JB. Atypical diabetes. American Diabetes Association, Arlington VA, 2018
19. Fajans SS, Bell GI. MODY. History, genetics, pathophysiology and clinical decision making. Diabetes Care 2011;34:1878–1884
20. Catalano P, Drago N, Amini S. Longitudinal changes in pancreatic beta-cell function and metabolic clearance rate of insulin in pregnant women with normal and abnormal glucose tolerance. Diabetes Care. 1998;21(3):403–408
21. Retnakaran R, Ying Q, Sermer M, et al. β-Cell function declines within the first year postpartum in women with recent glucose intolerance in pregnancy. Diabetes Care. 2010;33:1798–1804

3

Making the diagnosis of diabetes

Early diagnosis of diabetes is key to preventing the development of complications. This is especially important in the types of diabetes that present insidiously with long asymptomatic periods, such as type 2. Indeed, 50% of people with type 2 diabetes already have evidence of vascular disease at the time of diagnosis.

As described previously, diabetes is a group of metabolic disorders characterised by inappropriate hyperglycaemia that causes chronic microvascular, neuropathic and/or macrovascular disease. In determining diagnostic criteria, the difficult task has been to define exactly what constitutes 'inappropriate hyperglycaemia'. Our current diagnostic criteria are based on the decision to define inappropriate glycaemia as the level of glycaemia that puts a person at risk of developing retinopathy. However, it has not been possible to determine a measure of hyperglycaemia that best reflects this risk. Consequently, several diagnostic criteria exist for establishing the diagnosis of diabetes: a fasting blood glucose (FBG), an oral glucose tolerance test (OGTT) and haemoglobin A_{1c} (HbA$_{1c}$).

CRITERIA FOR THE DIAGNOSIS OF DIABETES

The American Diabetes Association has defined the following as criteria for the diagnosis of diabetes:[1]

1. FBG ≥ 7.0 mmol/L (126 mg/dL)
    Normal FBG is less than 5.6 mmol/L (100 mg/dL); a person with an FBG between 5.6 mmol/L (100 mg/dL) and 6.9 mmol/L (125 mg/dL) has 'impaired fasting glucose' (IFG).[1]

2. Random blood sugar test or OGTT following a 75-g glucose challenge ≥ 11 mmol/L (200 mg/dL)
    Normal blood sugar following a 75-g glucose challenge is less than 7.8 mmol/L (140 mg/dL); a person with a blood glucose between 7.8 mmol/L (140 mg/dL) and 11 mmol/L (199 mg/dL) following a glucose challenge has 'impaired glucose tolerance' (IGT).

3. HbA$_{1c}$ ≥ 48 mmol/mol (6.5%)[2]
    Those with an HbA$_{1c}$ between 39 mmol/mol (5.7%) and 47 mmol/mol (6.4%) are categorised as having 'pre-diabetes' (also called 'dysglycaemia' or 'borderline diabetes').

Of note, all the above blood tests should be done using venous plasma glucose (i.e. drawing the patient's blood). Basing a new diagnosis of diabetes on results from hand-held blood glucose meters or point-of-care HbA$_{1c}$ machines is not acceptable.

It is important to understand that, while these tests are relatively specific, none are particularly sensitive: there is a 20% false negative and false positive rate when an FBG or OGTT is used, while a positive HbA$_{1c}$ is 98.9% specific, but only 44.3% sensitive.[3] Thus, for a definitive diagnosis of diabetes, any positive test should be confirmed by a second test – preferably a repeat of the same test. If results are available from two different tests and one is positive and the other negative, the positive test should be repeated for diagnostic confirmation.[4] Only if a patient has a positive test and is obviously symptomatic (e.g. thirst, urinary frequency) is a confirmation test not required.

It is also important to understand that there is not perfect concordance between the three tests.[3,5–8] This is because each test reflects a different pathophysiological mechanism of abnormal glucose homeostasis.[9–11] As individuals have unique sets of pathologies contributing to their hyperglycaemia, it is not surprising that in one person one diagnostic test may be positive (e.g. an FBG) while another may be negative (e.g. HbA$_{1c}$).

For the same reason, each diagnostic test will identify a different set of individuals at risk for diabetes, and there is ongoing debate in the literature as to which should be the screening test of choice. A number of comparative studies looking at HbA$_{1c}$, FBG and OGTT have been done. These have produced some findings worth noting.

- Epidemiological studies carried out in the general population demonstrate that using the diagnostic criterion of HbA$_{1c}$ identifies one-third fewer cases of new diabetes than using an FBG.[3,12] Using FBG identifies about 50% more as having diabetes, while a combined FBG and 2-hour postprandial check (i.e. OGTT) will identify about 90% more as having diabetes.[13]
- HbA$_{1c}$ levels can vary in patients with certain anaemias, haemoglobinopathies or medical conditions with abnormal red cell turnover such as pregnancy, recent blood loss or transfusion. Notable differences in the normal distribution of HbA$_{1c}$ in relation to actual blood glucose levels have also been found across ethnic groups.[5,14] Using HbA$_{1c}$ to screen for type 2 diabetes in Asian Americans and Pacific Islanders misses 60% of the new diagnoses made when using an FBG and/or OGTT.[9,15]
- A positive OGTT/IGT is a stronger predictor of mortality and cardiovascular risk than a positive FBG or HbA$_{1c}$.[16,17]
- One of the advantages of using the HbA$_{1c}$ is that it has less day-to-day variability. However, as it is a measure of average blood sugar, it provides little information on pathophysiological processes contributing to the diabetes.[18] The OGTT is considered a better tool for identifying subjects with β-cell failure than is the HbA$_{1c}$.[19] When subjects without diabetes (defined as HbA$_{1c}$ < 39 mmol/mol [5.7%]) were stratified according to OGTT results, those with IFG

and/or IGT had a marked decrease in β-cell function compared with subjects with normal glucose tolerance, while subjects with pre-diabetes based on an HbA$_{1c}$ of 40–47 mmol/mol (5.7–6.4%) and a positive IFG and/or IGT had a further decrease in β-cell function. Because β-cell dysfunction is the principal factor responsible for the development and progression of type 2 diabetes, some authors recommend performing an OGTT for the assessment of β-cell health and better identification of subjects at increased risk for the development of type 2 diabetes.

SCREENING: TESTING FOR DIABETES IN ASYMPTOMATIC PATIENTS

Adults

Screening should begin at age 45. Testing should also be considered for adults who are younger than 45 years of age who are overweight or obese (BMI ≥ 25 kg/m^2) and have one or more additional risk factors for diabetes,[1–4] which include

- physical inactivity
- first-degree relative with diabetes
- high-risk race/ethnicity (e.g. African American, Latino, Native American, Asian American, Pacific Islander, Maori)
- women with a history of gestational diabetes or who have had a baby > 4.1 kg (9 lb)
- HDL < 0.9 mmol/L (35 mg/dL) and/or triglyceride level > 2.8 mmol/L (250 mg/dL)
- women with polycystic ovarian syndrome
- a clinical presentation associated with insulin resistance (morbid obesity, acanthosis nigricans)
- evidence of cardiovascular disease (e.g. hypertension, heart attack, stroke, peripheral vascular disease)
- long-term steroid or anti-psychotic use

Children and young adults

Testing should be considered for children and young adults who are overweight (BMI > 80th percentile for age; weight for height > 85th percentile;

or weight > 120% of ideal weight) plus any two of the following risk factors:[1–4]

- family history of type 2 diabetes in a first- or second-degree relative
- race/ethnicity (Native American, African American, Latino, Asian American, Pacific Islander, Maori)
- signs of insulin resistance or conditions associated with insulin resistance (acanthosis nigricans, hypertension, dyslipidaemia, polycystic ovarian syndrome or birth weight small for gestational age)
- maternal history of diabetes or gestational diabetes during child's gestation

Testing should begin at age 10 or at the onset of puberty if this occurs prior to age 10.

In general, if a person's screening test is negative, repeat screening is recommended every 3 years.[1]

MANAGEMENT FOLLOWING A POSITIVE TEST

Once a diagnosis of diabetes has been made, it is important that a full cardiovascular risk assessment and appropriate cardiovascular and glycaemic management follow. These are covered in detail in later chapters. In addition, microvascular screening programmes (retinal photography, renal function, foot checks) should be commenced.

Identifying a person with IFG or IGT is important as it signifies a person who not only is at a higher risk for developing diabetes but also has a higher cardiovascular risk. Of note, IGT is more strongly associated with cardiovascular events, cardiovascular mortality and progression on to diabetes than IFG.[13]

The progression to type 2 diabetes in individuals with pre-diabetes can be delayed by several years when they are treated with intensive lifestyle modification and/or pharmacological agents. Lifestyle modification and metformin can reduce the incidence of type 2 diabetes within 3 years by 58% and 38%, respectively.[20] Disappointingly, despite this opportunity for prevention, only 3.4% of individuals with pre-diabetes are aware of their diagnosis, suggesting that providers do not emphasise the importance of managing pre-diabetes with their patients.[21]

SUMMARY

- Diabetes is a group of metabolic disorders characterised by inappropriate hyperglycaemia.
- Three diagnostic criteria are currently being used to define a diagnosis of diabetes: fasting blood glucose (FBG), oral glucose tolerance test (OGTT) and haemoglobin A_{1c} (HbA_{1c}).
- All of the diagnostic tests are relatively specific; none are particularly sensitive. To make a definitive diagnosis of diabetes, any positive test must be repeated to confirm the diagnosis.
- Each diagnostic test reflects a different pathophysiologic mechanism of abnormal glucose homeostasis, so a person can test simultaneously positive for one test and negative for another.
- As diabetes can have an insidious onset, recommendations for screening the general population have been established.
- Early introduction of lifestyle changes and/or medication for a person with pre-diabetes can delay the onset of diabetes.

NOTES

1 Of note, other diabetes organisations including the World Health Organisation define IFG as from 6.1 mmol/L (110 mg/dL) to 6.9 mmol/L (125 mg/dL).

2 New Zealand chooses to use the diagnostic criterion of $HbA_{1c} \geq 50$ mmol/mol.[2]

REFERENCES

1. American Diabetes Association. Classification and diagnosis of diabetes: standards of medical care in diabetes – 2019. Diabetes Care. 2019;42(suppl1): S13–S28

2. New Zealand Society for the Study of Diabetes. Position statement on the diagnosis of, and screening for, type 2 diabetes, September 2011. 2011. Available at https://www.nzssd.org.nz/hba1c

3. Carson AP, Reynolds K, Fonseca VA, Munter P. Comparison of A1c and fasting glucose

criteria to diagnose diabetes among US adults. Diabetes Care. 2010;33:95–97

4. American Diabetes Association. Diagnosis and classification of diabetes. Diabetes Care. 2014;37(suppl 1): S81–S90

5. Christensen DL, Witte DR, Kaduka L, et al. Moving to an A1c-based diagnosis of diabetes has a different impact on prevalence in different ethnic groups. Diabetes Care. 2010;33:580–582

6. Kramer CK, Araneta MR, Barrett-Connor E. A1c and diabetes diagnosis: the Rancho Bernardo Study. Diabetes Care. 2010;33:101–103

7. Lorenzo C, Haffner SM. Performance characteristics of the new definition of diabetes: the Insulin Resistance Atherosclerosis Study. Diabetes Care. 2010;33:335–337

8. van't Reit E, Alssema M, Rijkelijkhuizen JM, et al. Relationship between A1c and glucose levels in the general Dutch population: the New Hoorn Study. Diabetes Care. 2010;33:61–66

9. Laakso M, Zilinskaite J, Hansen T, et al. Insulin sensitivity, insulin release and glucagon-like peptide-1 levels in persons with impaired fasting glucose and/or impaired glucose tolerance in the EUGENE2 study. Diabetologia. 2008;51:502–511

10. Nathan DM, Davidson MB, DeFronzo RA, et al. Impaired fasting glucose and impaired glucose tolerance: implications for care. Diabetes Care. 2007;30:753–759

11. Abdul-Ghani MA, Tripathy D, DeFronzo RA. Contributions of β-cell dysfunction and insulin resistance to the pathogenesis of impaired glucose tolerance and impaired fasting glucose. Diabetes Care. 2006;29:1130–1139

12. Lorenzo C, Wagenknecht LE, Hanley AJG, et al. A1c between 5.7 and 6.4% as a marker for identifying pre-diabetes, insulin sensitivity and secretion, and cardiovascular risk factors. Diabetes Care. 2010;33:2104–2109

13. Cederberg H, Saukkonen T, Laakso M, et al. Post-challenge glucose, A1c, and fasting glucose as predictors of type 2 diabetes and cardiovascular disease. Diabetes Care. 2010;33:2077–2083

14. Anand SS, Razak F, Vuksan V, et al. Diagnostic strategies to detect glucose intolerance in a multi-ethnic population. Diabetes Care. 2003;26:290–296

15. Araneta MR, Grandinetti A, Chang HK. A1c and diabetes diagnosis Among Filipino Americans, Japanese Americans, and Native Hawaiians. Diabetes Care. 2010; 33:2626–2628

16. International Expert Committee. International expert committee report on the role of the A1c assay in the diagnosis of diabetes. Diabetes Care. 2009;32:1327–1334

17. Novoa FJ, Boronat M, Saavedra, et al. Differences in cardiovascular risk factors, insulin resistance, and insulin secretion in individuals with normal glucose tolerance and in subjects with impaired glucose regulation: the Telde Study. Diabetes Care. 2005;28:2388–2393

18. Bonora E, Tuomilehto J. The pros and cons of diagnosing diabetes with A1c. Diabetes Care. 2011;34(suppl 2):S184–S190

19. Kanat M, Winnier D, Norton L, et al. The relationship between β-cell function and glycated haemoglobin. Diabetes Care. 2011;34:1006–1010

20. Diabetes Prevention Program Research Group. Within-trial cost-effectiveness of lifestyle intervention or metformin for the primary prevention of type 2 diabetes. Diabetes Care. 2003;26:2518–2523

21. Karve A, Hayward RA. Prevalence, diagnosis, and treatment of impaired fasting glucose and impaired glucose tolerance in nondiabetic US adults. Diabetes Care. 2010;33:2355–2359

4

Oral medications

The more that is understood about diabetes, the more it is seen as a heterogeneous group of diseases with a common expression (high blood sugars), with each type of diabetes having its own distinct set of pathophysiological mechanisms contributing to the shared expression of high blood sugars. With the discovery of each new contributing pathology, pharmaceutical companies have been quick to produce a medication that will assist with 'patching up' that particular pathology. Thus, each class of oral medication targets a different pathological mechanism in the glucose metabolic pathway. Numerous medications assist the pancreas with insulin production (sulfonylureas, glitinides); some medications suppress the production of glucose from the liver (biguinides) or absorption of glucose from the gut (α-glucosidase inhibitors); while others help to reduce insulin resistance (glitizones). The newest medications target the incretin system (the gliptins, GLP1 agonists) and the kidney (SGLT-2 inhibitors).

For many providers, the approach to introducing oral medications is much the same for everyone – a behaviour supported by patient management guidelines that are essentially prescriptive algorithms.[1,2] When only one or two drugs were available for diabetes management this 'one size fits all' approach was understandable. However, with the recognition that each person with diabetes has a unique set of underlying pathologies, along with our increasing ability to target these individual pathologies, a 'one size fits all' management regime is no longer necessarily appropriate. Increasingly, providers are recognising that only when medical management is appropriately tailored to each patient's underlying pathological processes will

optimal control of the disease be achieved.[3] How to establish each person's unique pathology is reviewed in Chapter 7, Considerations When Approaching Diabetes Management.

It is equally important to remember that considerations other than a person's pathophysiology should influence decisions around medical management. These include the extra-glycaemic effects that may contribute (negatively or positively) to long-term outcomes, medication safety profiles, medication expense, patient convenience and tolerability, and patient belief systems. Indeed, both the American Diabetes Association and the European Association for the Study of Diabetes have moved away from prescriptive management algorithms.[4,5] Rather, comprehensive reviews of all medical management options are provided, with an emphasis on the need to individualise choices based on clinical judgement and patient preference, noting that implementation of a successful management regime "will require thoughtful clinicians to integrate current evidence with other constraints and imperatives in the context of patient-specific factors".[4]

Below is a comprehensive list of the different oral medications,[1] their target/mode of action, side effects and contraindications, along with an indication of relative cost. Figure 4.1 provides not only an easy reference as to which pathology each oral medication targets, but an excellent pictorial representation of medications to assist patient understanding. After all, for patient preferences in medical management to be successfully established, each patient will need to gain a comprehensive understanding of all available medications.

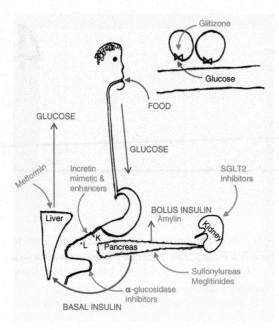

Figure 4.1 Primary pathological targets for each class of oral medication.

CLASS BIGUINIDE[2,4,6]

Compound Metformin

Route Oral. Available as short-acting, sustained-release and liquid formulations

Target Primary target – liver

Secondary targets – decreases insulin resistance

Action Decreases hepatic glucose output, primarily through inhibition of gluconeogenesis; clinically, decreases fasting glucose levels (note: 50% of the maximum dose will produce 80% of the maximum effect)

Side effects Common (minor in 30–50% of patients; significant in 5–15%); mostly gastric, with diarrhoea, nausea, vomiting, anorexia, gas, sometimes constipation, vitamin B_{12} deficiency. Side effects are dose-dependent, i.e. the side effects do not disappear unless you reduce the dose. For this reason, metformin should be started at the lowest dose (500 mg) with once a day dosing, increased to twice-daily dosing if the patient is tolerating it and then gradually stepped up to maximum dose (1500 mg twice daily). If the person develops side effects that are not tolerable, the dose should be dropped back in a stepwise fashion to a level that is tolerated

Contraindications Renal failure (recommendations differ between countries. The American Diabetes Association recommends discontinuation with estimated glomerular filtration rate (eGFR) < 30 mL/min per 1.73 m^2), cardiac or pulmonary insufficiency, liver disease, alcohol abuse and/or radiographic contrast agents

Advantages Weight-neutral, reduces cardiovascular events and mortality, excellent safety profile

Cost Very low (£)

CLASS SULFONYLUREA[4,7]

Compound First generation – chlorpropamide, tolazamide, tolbutamide

Second generation – glyburide, glipizide, gliclazide, glimepiride

Route Oral

Target Pancreas

Action Increases pancreatic insulin production independent of food intake

Side effects Hypoglycaemia, weight gain (≥ 2 kg after initiation), hypersensitivity reactions, hyponatraemia (rare)

Contraindications Insulin management, diabetes with pancreatic insufficiency, elderly, renal insufficiency

Disadvantages Weight gain, poor glycaemic durability

Cost Very low (£)

CLASS MEGLITINIDES[4,7]

Compound Repaglinide, nateglinide

Route Oral

Target Pancreas

Action Stimulates the pancreas to increase insulin secretion at time of food intake

Side effects Hypoglycaemia, weight gain (≥ 2 kg after initiation)

Contraindications Insulin use, diabetes with pancreatic insufficiency, elderly, renal insufficiency

Advantages Reduced hypoglycaemic episodes compared with sulfonylureas (as only active during ingestion of food)

Cost Low (££)

CLASS A-GLUCOSIDASE INHIBITORS[8]

Compound Acarbose, miglitol, voglibose

Route Oral

Target Gut wall

Action Targets postprandial sugars by inhibiting intestinal enzymes that cleave polysaccharides (complex carbohydrates) into monosaccharides (simple carbohydrates), thereby reducing gut absorption of glucose from ingested carbohydrates

Side effects Malabsorption-type symptoms: flatulence, diarrhoea, abdominal pain

Contraindications Insulin management, diabetes with pancreatic insufficiency

Cost Low (££)

CLASS THIAZOLIDINEDIONES (GLITAZONES)[9-11]

Compounds Pioglitazone, rosiglitazone

Route Oral

Target Activates the nuclear transcription factor PPAR-γ in muscle, adipose tissue and liver, increasing cellular responsiveness to insulin

Action Increases insulin sensitivity in liver and peripheral tissues; reduces triglycerides; reduces muscle and liver steatosis

Side effects Weight gain, fluid retention, peripheral oedema, osteoporosis, bone fractures, increases low-density lipoprotein (LDL). There are some inconclusive findings that suggest glitazones may be associated with an increased risk of developing bladder cancer

Contraindications New York Heart Association (NYHA) class III and IV heart failure, history of bladder cancer, history/risk of osteoporosis

Advantages Improves some lipid profiles (increases high-density lipoprotein (HDL), lowers triglycerides), possible delay in onset of microalbuminuria

Cost Moderate (£££)

CLASS DDP-4 INHIBITORS (GLIPTINS)[12]

Compounds Sitagliptin, vildagliptin, saxagliptin, linagliptin, alogliptin, anagliptin, tenegliptin

Route Oral

Target K and L cells in the gut endocrine system

Action K and L cells in the small intestine produce glucagon-like peptide 1 (GLP-1). GLP-1 is rapidly degraded by an enzyme, dipeptidyl-peptidase-4 (DDP-4). DDP-4 inhibitors prevent this degradation, prolonging the action of GLP-1. GLP-1 has four actions, it

- delays gastric emptying, minimising postprandial glucose load
- suppresses glucagon release (therefore suppressing hepatic gluconeogenesis)
- stimulates the pancreas to produce more insulin and
- stimulates the satiety centre in the central nervous system

Side effects Nausea, nasopharyngitis

Contraindications Renal insufficiency

Advantages Weight loss/neutrality, minimal risk of hypoglycaemia, reduces pancreatic lipotoxicity

Cost Moderate (£££)

CLASS GLP-1 RECEPTOR AGONIST (INCRETIN MIMETICS)[13]

Compounds Exenatide, liraglutide, lixisenatide, albiglutide, dulaglutide, semaglutide

Route Injectable; dosing is available as daily, twice daily or weekly

Target Gut endocrine system

Action Mimics the action of GLP-1 by activating GLP-1 receptors on pancreatic β-cells. GLP-1 agonists also increase β-cell growth. This enhances the four actions of GLP-1, it

- delays gastric emptying, minimising postprandial glucose load
- suppresses glucagon release (therefore suppressing hepatic gluconeogenesis)
- stimulates the pancreas to produce more insulin and
- stimulates the satiety centre in the central nervous system

Side effects Nausea, vomiting, diarrhoea, headache

Contraindications Renal insufficiency, type 1 diabetes or pancreatic insufficiency, pregnancy, lactation, gastroparesis

Advantages Weight loss, minimal risk of hypoglycaemia, reduces pancreatic lipotoxicity

Cost Very expensive (££££££)

CLASS SGLT-2 INHIBITORS (GLIFLOZINS)[14,15]

Compounds Dapagliflozin, canagliflozin, empagliflozin, ertugliflozin

Route Oral

Target Proximal tubule of the kidney

Action Blocks the sodium–glucose co-transporters (SGLT) in the proximal tubule, preventing the reabsorption of glucose back into the blood

Side effects Urinary tract/genital infections (more often in females), balanitis in males, normoglycaemic diabetic ketoacidosis (rare)

Contraindications Renal insufficiency (eGFR < 60 mL/min per 1.73 m^2), loop diuretic

Advantages Weight loss, decreased blood pressure, improved cardiovascular outcomes

Cost Expensive (££££)

CLASS DOPAMINE-2 AGONIST[16]

Compounds Bromocriptine

Route Oral

Target Central nervous system

Action Uncertain. As a dopamine agonist it is thought to moderate hypothalamic drive for increased plasma glucose, free fatty acids and triglycerides

Side effects Nausea

Contraindications Renal insufficiency (eGFR < 60 mL/min per 1.73 m^2), loop diuretic

Advantages Weight loss, minimal risk of hypoglycaemia

Cost Expensive (££££)

CLASS BILE ACID SEQUESTRANTS[4,17]

Compounds Colesevelam

Route Oral

Target Gall bladder

Action Bile acid sequestrant simultaneously lowering LDL and blood sugars. Mechanism for lowering blood sugars is not well understood

Side effects Mainly gastric, including dyspepsia, diarrhoea/constipation, flatulence. Raised triglycerides

Contraindications High triglycerides

Advantages Lowers LDL

Cost Moderately expensive (£££)

CLASS AMYLIN ANALOGUE[8]

Compounds Pramlintide

Route Injectable (subcutaneous)

Target Central nervous system receptors

Action Mimics amylin, a hormone that is co-secreted with insulin from the pancreatic β-cells, regulating the postprandial rate of glucose entry into the circulation – i.e. helps to manage postprandial blood sugars.

Side effects Nausea, hypoglycaemia

Cost Extremely expensive
(£££££££££
£££££££££££)

Many of the above medications have been combined into single tablets. Available drug combinations include:

Metformin + glipizide (Metaglip)
Metformin + glyburide (Glucovance)
Metformin + repaglinide (Prandimet)

Metformin + pioglitizone (Actoplus)
Metformin + rosiglitazone (Avandamet)

Metformin + sitagliptin (Janumet)
Metformin + alogliptin (Kazano)
Metformin + saxagliptin (Kombiglyze)
Metformin + linagliptin (Jentadueto)

Metformin + canagliflozin (Invokamet)
Metformin + dapagliflozin (Xigduo)
Metformin + empagliflozin (Synjardy)

Metformin + dapagliflozin + saxagliptin
  (Qtermet XR)

Glimepiride + rosiglitazone (Avandaryl)
Glimepiride + pioglitazone (Duetact)

Pioglitizone + alogliptin (Oseni)

Linagliptin + empagliflozin (Glyxambi)
Sitagliptin + simvastatin (Juvisync)

SUMMARY

- Each class of oral medications targets a different pathophysiological mechanism underlying diabetes.
- Choice of oral medication should be guided by a patient's underlying pathophysiology, as well as by effectiveness in lowering glucose, extra-glycaemic effects that may reduce long-term complications, contribution to cardiovascular risk reduction, medication safety profiles, tolerability and expense.

- Guidelines have been established to support medical management decision-making. However, these are becoming less prescriptive, acknowledging individual differences in underlying pathologies and patient preferences.

NOTE

1 Availability of medications differs between countries.

REFERENCES

1. Nathan DM, Buse JB, Davidson MB, et al. Management of hyperglycemia in type 2 diabetes: a consensus algorithm for the initiation and adjustment of therapy: a consensus statement from the American Diabetes Association and the European Association for the Study of Diabetes. Diabetes Care. 2006:29:1963–1972
2. New Zealand Guidelines Group. Guidance on the management of type 2 diabetes. In The New Zealand Primary Care Handbook 2011. New Zealand Ministry of Health, Wellington, 2011. Downloadable from www.nzgg.org.nz
3. Fowler MJ. Diabetes treatment: oral agents. Clin Diabetes. 2010;28:132–136
4. American Diabetes Association. Classification and diagnosis of diabetes: standards of medical care in diabetes – 2019. Diabetes Care. 2019;42(suppl1):S96–S102
5. Inzucchi SE, Bergenstal RM, Buse JB, et al. Management of hyperglycemia in type 2 diabetes: a patient-centred approach. Position statement of the American Diabetes Association (ADA) and the European Association for the Study of Diabetes (EASD). Diabetes Care. 2012;35:1364–1379
6. Bailey CJ, Turner RC. Metformin. N Engl J Med. 1996;334:574–579
7. Gangji AS, Cukierman T, Gerstein HC, et al. A systematic review and meta-analysis of hypoglycaemia and cardiovascular events: a comparison of glyburide with other secretagogues and with insulin. Diabetes Care. 2007:30:389–394
8. Fonseca VA. Clinical diabetes: translating research into practice. Saunders Elsevier, Philadelphia, 2006
9. Schwartz AV, Sellmeyer DE, Vittinghoff E, et al. Thiazolidinedione use and bone loss in older diabetic adults. J Clin Endocrinol Metab. 2006;91:3349–3354

10. Yki-Jarvinen H. Thiazolidinediones. N Engl J Med. 2004;351:1106–1118
11. Tang H, Shi W, Fu S, et al. Pioglitizone and bladder cancer risk: a systematic review and meta-analysis. Cancer Med. 2018;7:1070–1080
12. Gupta V, Kalra S. Choosing a gliptin. Indian J Endocrinol Metab. 2011;15:298–308
13. Ahren B, Holst JJ, Mari A. Characterization of GLP-1 effects on beta-cell function after meal ingestion in humans. Diabetes Care. 2003;26:2860–2864
14. Chao EC. SGLT-2 Inhibitors: a new mechanism for glycemic control. Clin Diabetes. 2014;32:4–11
15. Abdul-Ghani M, Del Prato S, Chilton R, et al. SGLT2 inhibitors and cardiovascular risk: lessons learned from the EMPA-REG OUTCOME study. Diabetes Care. 2016; 39(5):717–725
16. Shivaprasad C, Kalra S. Bromocriptine in type 2 diabetes mellitus. Indian J Endocrinol Metab. 2011;15(suppl):S17–S24
17. Fonseca VA, Handelsman Y, Staels B. Colesevelam lowers glucose and lipid levels in type 2 diabetes: the clinical evidence. Diabetes Obes Metab. 2010;12(5):384–392.

5

Insulins and insulin management

While one can think of oral medications as 'patching up' pathology, exogenous insulins are about *replacing* pathology; they replace the basal and bolus insulin secretion of the pancreas (see Figure 1.2).

If the blood glucose of a person without diabetes was checked upon waking it would be around 4 mmol/L (70 mg/dL). This fasting blood glucose reflects hepatic glucose secretion. If this person did not eat all day, the cells would continue to be supplied with glucose from the liver. Of course, as described earlier, this hepatic glucose is suitably matched by pancreatic insulin (basal insulin) to allow cellular blood glucose uptake. Thus, despite ongoing hepatic glucose supply, the blood sugars do not rise but essentially remain around 4 mmol/L (70 mg/dL).

If this person without diabetes should then eat, a spike will occur in the blood glucose secondary to ingested carbohydrates. Because the pancreas matches this glucose influx with a bolus of insulin, the blood glucose spike does not rise above 7.8 mmol/L (140 mg/dL) and the blood sugar returns to baseline relatively quickly – around 2–5 hours depending on the content of the food ingested.

In Figure 5.1, these two sources of glucose (hepatic and ingested) have been represented graphically over time (solid lines). As there are two 'types' of pancreatic insulin secretion (basal and bolus) to match the two sources of glucose, this graph can also be seen to represent (simplistically) insulin secretion over a 24-hour period (dotted lines).

Clearly, a person without diabetes has a perfect match between their physiologic blood glucose (solid lines) and their insulin secretion (the dotted lines). If they did not, they would experience hyperglycaemia (i.e. too little insulin relative to the blood glucose) and/or hypoglycaemia (i.e. too much insulin relative to the blood glucose). Thus, when introducing exogenous insulin with the objective of achieving tight glycaemic control in a person with diabetes, the goal is to match as closely as possible the physiologic glucose pattern of the person being treated.[1] Indeed, the driving force behind pharmaceutical companies' continually developing different

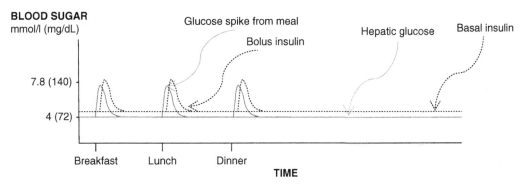

Figure 5.1 The physiologic pattern of blood glucose (solid lines) and insulin (dotted lines) secretion in a person without diabetes over a 24-hour period.

insulins and different insulin delivery systems is the desire to produce insulins with pharmacokinetic profiles that match physiologic blood glucose secretion as closely as possible.

Of note, it is important not to assume that everyone has the same physiologic glucose pattern. Each will be unique, as people skip meals, eat different foods or eat at different times of the day. Thus, before choosing an insulin regime for a patient, it is essential to determine the person's physiologic glucose pattern.

One of the ongoing debates in the management of people with type 2 diabetes is whether insulin should be introduced early in the progression of the disease or late. Until relatively recently, the introduction of insulin for someone with type 2 diabetes was considered a last resort after all else had failed. In part, this has been for historical reasons, with older, traditional insulins doing less well with matching normal physiologic glucose patterns and thereby increasing the risk of hypoglycaemia.[2–4] However, now that we recognise β-cell deterioration as a primary pathology contributing to disease progression in type 2 diabetes, insulin is being introduced earlier;[5] and with the development of analogue insulins, sophisticated insulin delivery systems and improved blood glucose monitoring abilities, a good physiologic match is achievable and the risk of hypoglycaemia relatively low.[2] Indeed, these advances in insulin management have reduced the rates of severe hypoglycaemia in type 1 diabetes despite a continual tightening of glycaemic control over recent years.[6]

Insulin may also have some advantages over oral medications: doses can be tailored to match individual needs,[7] it is relatively cheap, there is little to no intolerance and, other than the risk of hypoglycaemia, there are few adverse effects.[2] It is the only hypoglycaemic agent that reduces lipolysis and decreases free fatty acid concentrations in blood.[8] This improves insulin action and secretion,[7,9] reduces non-alcoholic steatohepatitis,[10] decreases LDL cholesterol and triglycerides and increases HDL cholesterol.[11]

The reasons most often given by providers who do not support early introduction of insulin include increased risk of hypoglycaemia, weight gain and a theoretical risk of cancer.[12] The threat of hypoglycaemia will always be a major barrier to optimising glycaemic control. However, as noted above, much of the support for arguments around increased

hypoglycaemia come from studies that have used traditional non-physiologic insulins. Weight gain is also associated more with non-physiologic insulin regimes.[13] This is due not only to the increased frequency of hypoglycaemia requiring carbohydrate intake for management, but also to the practice of prescribing regular in-between meal snacking to insure against hypoglycaemic episodes. While there appears to be an association of cancer with increased insulin levels (exogenous and/or endogenous), obesity with its associated cancer risk has been a major confounding factor. In the few studies where obesity has been controlled for, no conclusive evidence has been found to support the argument that exogenous insulin directly increases the risk of cancer.[14,15]

Resistance from patients is another reason given for the lack of early introduction. However, studies suggest that patients are actually 'psychologically insulin-receptive' when the topic is broached, and that clinical inertia is much more likely to be due to providers who are uncomfortable with insulin management.[4]

INSULIN PHARMACOKINETICS

The ability to mimic pancreatic function requires a long-acting basal insulin dosed to cover 24 hours and a short-acting bolus insulin that is physiologically active for short periods of time (2–4 hours). Despite this apparent need for just two types of insulin, there are many different exogenous insulins. This large array of available insulins is due to a number of reasons:

- A century of trying to develop insulins that closely mimic the basal and bolus profiles of pancreatic function. The early insulins, referred to as the 'traditional' insulins, are a less-than-ideal physiologic match as they are biphasic with basal and bolus components. The newer insulins are monophasic (hence the name 'analogue') and therefore more physiologic.
- There are three different pharmaceutical companies each producing both traditional and analogue insulins.
- The introduction of insulin mixes which combine basal and bolus insulins within the same vial. These were introduced to minimise the need for multiple shots. The basal component of all insulin mixes is neutral

protamine hagedorn (NPH)/isophane. The traditional insulin mix has a traditional bolus insulin combined with NPH, while the newer insulin mixes have an analogue bolus insulin combined with NPH. The basal and bolus components have been combined in different ratios, and the numbers included in the name of each insulin mix indicate the ratio of the basal and bolus components. For example, Humalog mix 25 is mixed in a ratio of 25% Humalog and 75% Humulin N, while Novomix 70/30 has 70% Novolin N with 30% Novorapid (Novolog).

Insulins are delivered either subcutaneously or inhaled. Tables 5.1, 5.2 categorise the available subcutaneous insulins according to which company produces them and whether they are traditional or analogue. Each insulin has a unique pharmacokinetic or action profile that includes either a basal component, a bolus component or, in the case of the traditional insulins, both basal and bolus components. The simplest way to approach insulin management is to determine which part of a person's physiologic insulin profile (basal versus bolus) you wish to replace and then select an insulin with a pharmacokinetic profile that has the best match.

The pharmacokinetic profile of each insulin is described below accompanied by a graphical representation of this profile. Of note, the pharmacokinetic profiles can vary between patients and, particularly in the case of the traditional insulins, they can vary on a day-to-day basis within the same patient.

Obviously, pharmacokinetic profiles of insulin mixes reflect the individual profiles of the basal and bolus insulin that have been included in the mix.

Most subcutaneous insulins are produced in a concentration of 100 units/mL and referred to as U-100. However, with the growing obesity epidemic and its accompanying insulin resistance, higher doses of insulin are being required.[16] To address the high insulin requirements, more concentrated formulations of insulin have been introduced. Eli Lilly was the first pharmaceutical company to develop one such insulin, Humulin R U-500. Other pharmaceutical companies are following suit. U-500 insulin is at the concentration of 500 units/mL, i.e. it contains the same number of units as U-100 insulin but in one-fifth of the volume; while U-200 insulin is at a concentration of 200 units/mL, i.e. it contains the same number of units as U-100 insulin in one-half of the volume.

Table 5.1 Exogenous subcutaneous insulin by pharmaceutical company: traditional insulins

Pharmaceutical company	Basal insulin (NPH/isophane)	Bolus insulin	Insulin mixes (NPH/isophane + traditional bolus)
Lilly	Humulin N	Humulin R (Regular)	Humulin 70/30; 50/50
Novo Nordisk	Novolin N (Protaphane)	Novolin R (Actrapid)	Novolin 70/30
Sanofi Aventis	–	–	–

Table 5.2 Exogenous subcutaneous insulin by pharmaceutical company: analogue insulins

Pharmaceutical company	Basal insulin	Bolus insulin	Insulin mixes (NPH/isophane + analogue bolus)
Lilly	–	Lispro (Humalog)	Humalog mix (multiple combinations available)
Novo Nordisk	Detemir (Levemir)	Aspart (Novolog/Novorapid)	Novolog mix (multiple combinations available)
	Degludec (Tresiba)	Fiasp (Aspart rapid acting)	
Sanofi Aventis	Glargine (Lantus)	Glulisine (Apidra)	–

Traditional subcutaneous insulins

Basal Neutral protamine hagedorn (NPH)/isophane

Pharmacokinetic profile Biphasic with a basal and bolus component, with the basal component more prominent (Figure 5.2). Historically, both components were taken advantage of by dosing two-thirds in the morning and one-third in the evening. The intention was for the peak of the morning dose to coincide with lunchtime. Today, NPH is mostly used as a basal insulin, dosed to take advantage of the basal component by giving two to three equal doses evenly across the day

Onset of action 1–2 hours

Action peak (bolus component) 4–6 hours

Duration of action (basal component) 12–16 hours

Advantages Inexpensive (£)

Disadvantages Biological variability of 50%. This variability contributes to increased hypoglycaemia with tightening up of control. The variability is partly due to this being a cloudy insulin; each time it is used it has to be mixed, and it is impossible to ensure an entirely homogenous mixture after each mixing

Bolus Humulin R, Novolin R

Pharmacokinetic profile Biphasic with a basal and bolus component, with the bolus component more prominent (Figure 5.3). Most often used as a bolus insulin for mealtime cover, taking advantage of the bolus component

Onset of action 30–60 minutes

Action peak (bolus component) 2–4 hours

Duration of action (basal component) 6–8 hours

Advantages Inexpensive (£)

Disadvantages Poor physiologic match to meal-time blood sugar spikes as well as a 30-minute delay in the onset of action. To obtain the best physiologic match the insulin should be given 30 minutes prior to a meal. Biological variability of 50%, contributing to increased hypoglycaemia and weight gain. Does not lend itself to carbohydrate counting

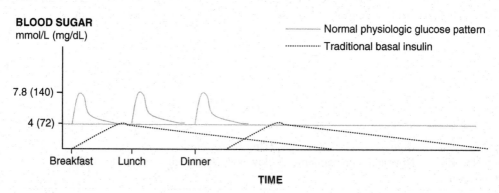

Figure 5.2 The pharmacokinetic profile of traditional basal insulin.

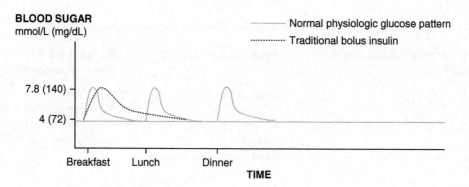

Figure 5.3 The pharmacokinetic profile of traditional bolus insulin.

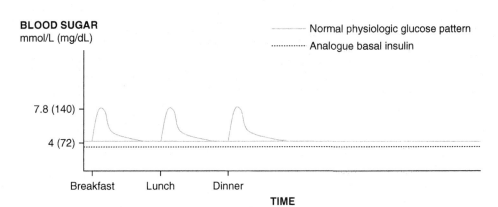

Figure 5.4 The pharmacokinetic profile of analogue basal insulin.

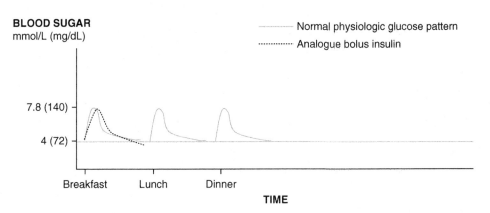

Figure 5.5 The pharmacokinetic profile of analogue bolus insulin.

Analogue subcutaneous insulins

Basal Glargine (U-100 and U-300), detemir, degludec (U-100 and U-200)

Pharmacokinetic profile Analogue insulin with a basal component only (Figure 5.4)

Onset of action 2 hours

Action peak (bolus component) Minimal to none

Duration of action (basal component)

Glargine ≥ 24 hours
Detemir 14–16 hours. Recommended twice-daily dosing, but often used as once-daily dosing
Degludec – an ultra-long acting basal insulin with a duration of action of > 42 hours

Advantages Glargine and detemir have a good physiologic match with only 20% biological variability. This reduces blood glucose variability, allowing for tighter control with fewer hypoglycaemic episodes.[17,18] When compared with NPH there is little to no increased risk of weight gain in people with type 1 diabetes and a lower risk of weight gain in people with type 2 diabetes

Disadvantage Expensive (££–££££)

Bolus Lispro (U-100 and U-200), aspart, glulisine

Pharmacokinetic profile Analogue insulin with a bolus component only (Figure 5.5)

Onset of action Lispro, glulisine and aspart 5–10 minutes

Action Peak 30–60 minutes

Duration of action 3–4 hours

Advantages The analogue bolus insulins have a relatively close physiologic match for mealtime blood glucose spikes. This allows for tighter control with fewer hypoglycaemic events. Can be used to match insulin to carbohydrate intake ('carb counting') and to correct high blood sugars

Disadvantage Moderately expensive (£–£££)

Analogue inhaled insulins

Bolus Afrezza

Pharmacokinetic profile Analogue insulin with a bolus component only

Onset of action Immediate (< 1 minute)

Action Peak 12–15 minutes

Duration of action 1.5–3 hours

Advantages Rapid onset of action with excellent match to physiologic glucose spike

Disadvantages Single-use capsules with pre-set doses in increments of 2 units limiting ability to match insulin dose to carbohydrate intake. Contraindicated in people with chronic lung disease and tobacco use. Regular pulmonary function testing recommended. Long-term pulmonary safety unknown. Expensive (£££)

INSULIN DELIVERY

Injectable insulin should be placed subcutaneously. This is done either by syringe, insulin pen or continuous subcutaneous insulin infusion (CSII) – more commonly known as the insulin pump.

Subcutaneous syringes Syringes (Figure 5.6) provide the least accurate delivery; the insulin is drawn up manually from a vial, allowing opportunity for air bubbles; the tiny markings on the outside of the syringe are difficult for many to see, increasing the risk of incorrect dosing; and the needles are long, increasing the likelihood that the insulin will not be deposited subcutaneously. Magnifiers that clip onto the side of the syringe are available.

- Syringes come in different sizes:
    - 3 mL (3/10 cc) to deliver a maximum of 30 units. The markings on the outside do allow for the delivery of half-unit increments.
    - 5 mL (½ cc) to deliver a maximum of 50 units.
    - 10 mL (1 cc) to deliver a maximum of 100 units.

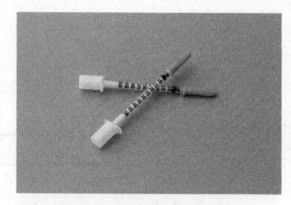

Figure 5.6 Subcutaneous insulin syringes.

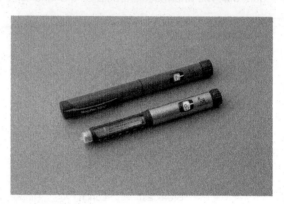

Figure 5.7 Insulin pens.

- The syringes are packaged in bags of ten. A box of syringes can contain five bags (50 syringes) or ten bags (100 syringes).

Insulin pens Insulin pens (Figure 5.7) allow a person to 'dial up' the number of units needed, increasing the ease and accuracy of delivery. Some pens can measure up insulin in increments of half-units.

Most pens need to be manually loaded with a 3 mL cartridge of insulin (total of 300 units). Insulin cartridges must be paired up with insulin pens made by the same pharmaceutical company.

Some companies produce disposable insulin pens that come pre-loaded with the 300 units of insulin. Novo Nordisk produces a 'memory' pen that stores information about past doses taken.

Should the patient overshoot the desired number of units when dialling up, the dial can be wound backwards to the desired number of units before insulin delivery without any risk of overdelivering insulin. Magnifiers that fit over the window indicating the number of units being dialled are available for some pens.

Insulin pen needles All insulin pens, disposable or non-disposable, require needles to be prescribed separately (Figure 5.8). Needles come in different sizes (4 mm, 5 mm, 8 mm, 12.7 mm). However, as the thickness of skin is the same in thin and obese patients, and the insulin needs to be placed subcutaneously, a 4-mm needle is recommended for everyone. If an injection is too deep, the insulin is absorbed faster, possibly causing hypoglycaemia, and it has a shorter pharmacokinetic profile.[19]

Continuous subcutaneous insulin infusion (insulin pump) The insulin pump (Figure 5.9) is a small computerised device approximately 9 cm (3.5 inches) × 5 cm (2 inches) in size. It is worn externally, either clipped onto the waistband or belt or put in a pocket. It is connected subcutaneously by tubing and an infusion set. The insulin pump contains an analogue bolus insulin and delivers the basal component of management via a continuous 24-hour drip. One advantage of insulin delivery via

an insulin pump is the ability to alter the rate of basal insulin delivery at any time to accommodate decreased or increased insulin needs, such as with exercise or illness.

At mealtimes a bolus of insulin can be delivered with the push of a button or touch of the insulin pump screen. The insulin pump is programmed to calculate insulin doses based on a person's blood sugar and the carbohydrate content of a meal.

Insulin delivery via an insulin pump is around 5% variable, allowing tighter control with little increase in the risk of hypoglycaemia. Some insulin pumps come with integrated continuous glucose monitoring systems (CGMS) which continually feed blood glucose information to the insulin pump, and this in turn automatically adjusts insulin delivery. For more information on CGMS see Chapter 8, Glycaemic Management.

INSULIN DOSE CALCULATIONS

The starting point for calculating insulin doses, regardless of type of diabetes, is a formula that estimates a person's total daily dose of insulin (TDDI). However, there are some nuances in the insulin needs of children and adults with type 1 diabetes that complicate the instructions, putting them outside the scope of this manual. The following instructions for insulin dosing are for adults with type 2 diabetes.

Depending on which resource used, there is some variability in the formula. The formula we will use for calculating the TDDI is

$$TDDI = 0.8 \text{ units insulin} \times \text{patient weight (kg)/day}$$

For example, for an 80-kg man

$$TDDI = 0.8 \text{ units of insulin} \times 80 \text{ kg/day}$$

$$= 64 \text{ units of insulin/day}$$

As this is the TDDI, it includes both the basal and bolus insulin requirements. In a person with type 2 diabetes, the basal component constitutes around 40–60% of the TDDI. Thus, if one were to initiate a basal insulin dose that is 30% of the calculated TDDI there would be little risk of the person experiencing hypoglycaemia.

Further reassurance is gained by knowing that this formula calculates the amount of insulin

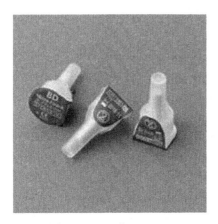

Figure 5.8 Insulin pen needles.

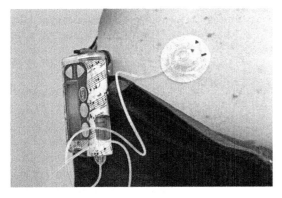

Figure 5.9 Subcutaneous insulin pump.

required by a person who is insulin-sensitive, which means that for obese, insulin-resistant people (i.e. those with type 2 diabetes) the formula *underestimates* the TDDI. Thus, using 30% of the TDDI as the starting dose is very unlikely to result in hypoglycaemia.

Calculating a starting basal insulin dose for a person with type 2 diabetes

1. Calculate TDDI.
2. Calculate 30% of the TDDI as your *starting* basal dose.
   a. If traditional basal insulin is being used, usual practice is to divide the starting dose evenly into two and have the patient take one dose in the morning and the second in the evening. A more physiologic delivery can be achieved by dividing the starting dose into three and delivering the insulin three times a day (breakfast, lunch and dinner).
   b. If analogue basal insulin is being used, have the patient choose a time of day when they can reliably take the shot at the same time each day.
3. Instruct the patient to monitor fasting blood sugars.
4. Escalate insulin dose by 10% every 2–3 days until goal waking blood sugars are achieved. Note that if the person's blood sugars have been very poorly controlled for a period of time (> 12 weeks), the titration should be done more gradually to prevent the person from experiencing symptoms of hypoglycaemia as blood sugars approach the normal range.
5. You may choose to have the patient monitor blood sugars and adjust their own insulin doses accordingly. Indeed, research has demonstrated that patients achieve more efficient insulin titration than providers.[20] See Patient Handouts 5 and 6, 'Monitoring Your Blood Sugar's, for patient instructions on insulin titration.

Remember:
- The initial starting dose calculated will be an underestimate of the patient's needs. Thus, the risk of a hypoglycaemic event is essentially

zero. If hypoglycaemia occurs, this should immediately raise a red flag as to whether the person has insulin resistance, i.e. type 2 diabetes.
- Be sure to review the section at the end of this chapter on important information to review with patients using insulin.

Calculating a starting dose for meal-time insulin for a person with type 2 diabetes

Calculating a starting dose for mealtime insulin uses the calculated TDDI, the '500 rule' and relies on the assumption that the average adult eats 50 g carbohydrate per meal. These calculations can be used for both analogue and traditional bolus insulins although, as noted above, the analogue insulin profiles will provide a superior physiologic match to a person's postprandial blood sugars.

Dividing 500 by TDDI provides a person's carbohydrate ratio, i.e. how many grams of carbohydrate need to be consumed to match 1 unit of insulin.

For example, for the 80-kg man

$$TDDI = 0.8 \text{ units} \times 80 \text{ kg/day}$$
$$= 64 \text{ units a day}$$

Apply the '500 rule':

$$\frac{500}{TDDI} = \frac{500}{64}$$
$$\approx 8 \text{ g}$$

Thus, 1 unit of insulin is needed for every 8 g carbohydrate consumed.

Assuming the average adult meal contains 50 g carbohydrate, a safe *starting* mealtime dose of insulin for this 80-kg man would be

$$\frac{50 \text{ g carbohydrate meal}}{8 \text{ g per unit of insulin}} \approx 6 \text{ units insulin per meal}$$

In summary, a person who weighs 80 kg whose basal insulin needs are around 40 units (following titration up from a starting basal dose of 21 units) can be started with a set mealtime bolus of 6 units of insulin.

Of note, most adults eat more than 50 g carbohydrates per meal. So, once again, basing the calculation of the mealtime dose on a 50-g carbohydrate meal minimises the risk of post-meal hypoglycaemia. Obviously, subsequent up-titration of the mealtime dose to match food intake will be needed.

It is very important to understand that there is a tight relationship between the basal insulin dose and the mealtime dose as both are calculated using TDDI. This means that if a person's basal insulin dose increases, it necessarily follows that the TDDI increases, which in turn means the carbohydrate ratio will decrease and the mealtime insulin dose increase. Table 5.3 illustrates this tight relationship.

Note that it is a rare for a person to need more than 20 units of bolus insulin with a meal. Indeed, if they are needing more than 20 units of insulin with each meal their eating habits should be reviewed (see Chapter 9, Lifestyle Management).

Based on the above, the expectation is that a person taking more than 20 units of insulin with each meal must have a basal insulin dose of 200 units or more. If their basal insulin is not well into the hundreds, then either

- there is an incorrect relationship between their basal insulin dose and their bolus insulin dose, i.e. the basal is too low so that the person comes into each meal with a high blood sugar; the large mealtime bolus is then accommodating both mealtime carbohydrate intake and a 'correction' for the high blood sugar. A person with this kind of basal/bolus mismatch usually presents with a high HbA$_{1c}$ but is experiencing recurrent post-meal hypoglycaemic episodes

or

- the person is grossly overeating (meals are 80–120 g carbs) and they are gaining weight.

Remember:

- Everyone using mealtime insulin should be provided with accurate information on how different foods affect blood sugars differently, and how different types of foods can be combined to optimise the match between postprandial blood glucose rise and insulin pharmacokinetics (see Chapter 9, Lifestyle Management).

Carbohydrate counting

For those with type 2 diabetes, good blood sugar control can generally be obtained with a fixed mealtime dose of insulin. However, some may wish to fine-tune their blood glucose management by calculating the carbohydrate content of each meal (in grams) and using their carbohydrate ratio (see above) to calculate the insulin dose required for the meal. Certainly, anyone managing their diabetes with an insulin pump should be encouraged to 'carb count' each meal.

Packaged foods are legally required to document the grams of carbohydrate per serving. Non-packaged foods such as fruit and vegetables obviously do not come with this information, but multiple resources are available to assist with carbohydrate counting:

- Reference books, available at any bookstore or on the web. One of the best is *Calorie Fat and Carbohydrate Counter* by Allan Borushek (Family Health Publications, 2020). www.CalorieKing.com

Table 5.3 Relationship between basal and bolus insulin doses

Total daily dose of insulin (TDDI)	Basal dose (based on 60% TDDI)	Calculated carbohydrate ratio (500/TDDI)	Number of units needed for 50-g carbohydrate meal	Number of units needed for 80-g carbohydrate meal
64 units	≈40 units	1:8 g	6 units	10 units
80 units	≈50 units	1:6 g	8 units	13 units
125 units	≈80 units	1:4 g	12 units	20 units
175 units	≈110 units	1:3 g	16 units	26 units

- American Diabetes Association website.
- Carbohydrate counting apps for phones/computers
- Some electronic food scales have programs that calculate the carbohydrate content of the food being weighed.

Calculating a correction factor

A correction factor, also known as an insulin sensitivity factor or sliding scale, allows a person to calculate insulin doses to correct a high (or low) blood sugar. This is not difficult to do. Anyone who can manage their pocket change is more than capable of using a correction factor.

There are a number of advantages to teaching this skill to people with type 2 diabetes who are using a bolus insulin:

- It introduces flexibility in eating without worsening blood sugar control and reduces the guilt associated with eating. If a person wishes to 'splurge' at a social event or eat a snack between meals, there is no need to feel guilty about the resultant high blood sugar as they know they can simply correct it at the next meal.
- Being able to correct a blood sugar empowers the patient; it provides them with a skill that puts them in full control of their blood sugars.
- It necessarily requires a pre-meal blood sugar check, i.e. ensures that a person is regularly checking their blood sugars prior to delivering insulin.
- It reduces the risk of post-meal hypoglycaemia or hyperglycaemia.

Calculating the correction factor uses the TDDI and the '100 rule' (or the '1800 rule' in countries where blood sugar is measured in mg/dL).[1] Dividing 100 by TDDI provides the number of mmol/L that 1 unit of insulin will drop blood glucose.

For example, for a 72-kg man

$$TDDI = 0.8 \text{ units} \times 72 \text{ kg/day}$$
$$= 57 \text{ units a day}$$

Apply the '100 rule':

$$\frac{100}{TDDI} = \frac{100}{57}$$
$$\approx 2$$

Thus, 1 unit of analogue insulin will bring the blood sugar down by 2 mmol/L; i.e. if a person has a blood glucose of 12 mmol/L and they take 3 units of bolus insulin, their blood sugar will be 6 mmol/L 3 hours later.

Remember:

- An analogue bolus insulin lasts for approximately 3 hours, so a person should not be re-correcting their blood sugars within 3 hours of a previous correction. The only time this can be done is when they have been taught how to calculate 'insulin on board'.
- Using a traditional bolus insulin for correcting blood sugars is possible. However, because of its 6- to 8-hour pharmacokinetic profile, it will take twice as long to reach the desired glycaemic target and be less convenient for recurrent corrections.

ESSENTIAL TEACHING POINTS

The following are essential teaching points to review with every patient when initiating insulin.

- Priming the needle (Figure 5.10). Anyone using an insulin pen should be instructed to fill the needle with insulin prior to dialling up their planned insulin dose. A needle is hollow and, depending on the size of the needle, it holds 2–4 units of insulin. If the needle is not 'primed' prior to dialling up the desired dose,

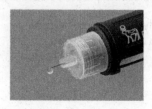

Figure 5.10 Priming the needle should be done before every insulin injection.

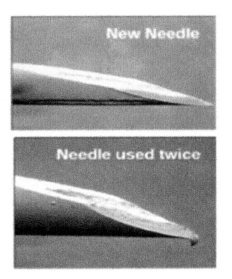
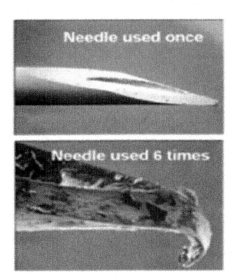

Figure 5.11 Deterioration of insulin needles with use.

the patient will not receive their full dose; they will be 2–4 units short.

- Safe needle disposal. Used needles are considered to be infectious medical waste and should be disposed of according to the local legal requirements.
- Changing needles (Figure 5.11). Insulin needles should be changed following each use. This minimises the risk of infection. The needles also deteriorate with each use, and the deposition of metal microfibres may possibly contribute to the development of lipodystrophy.
- Rotation of shots (Figures 5.12 and 5.13). Injecting insulin into the same area causes lipodystrophic or lipohypertrophic changes to subcutaneous fat. Aside from being unsightly, any insulin delivered into lipohypertrophic areas has reduced and more unpredictable absorption.[21] Patients should be encouraged to rotate their shots (or insulin infusion set if on an insulin pump), using arms, legs, abdomen and gluteals.
- Avoiding mixing insulins. Long-acting analogue insulins cannot be mixed with any other insulin. A general rule of thumb is to instruct the patient to rotate the delivery of the long-acting analogue insulin on one side of the body, and rotate the rapid-acting insulin on the opposite side of the body.
- Understanding the symptoms and management of hypoglycaemia.

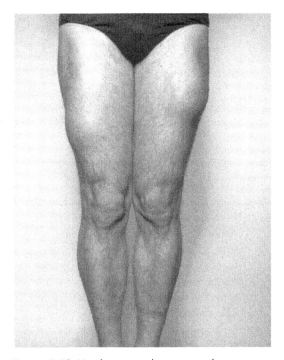

Figure 5.12 Lipohypertrophy occurs when injections are repeatedly given in the same place on the body.

- Safe storage. Insulin not being used should be stored in the refrigerator. Insulin pens or vials of insulin being used should be kept at room temperature.

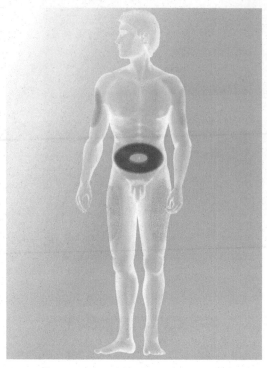

Figure 5.13 Recommended insulin injection sites. To avoid lipodystrophy or lipohypertrophy, insulin delivery should be rotated between the trunk, buttocks and extremities.

- Each insulin has its own pharmacokinetic profile. However, this profile can vary depending on the insulin's reliability, and on individual patient responses.
- Insulin comes in concentrations of U-100, U-200 and U-500.
- Delivery of insulin is either subcutaneous or inhaled.
- The starting point for all insulin dose calculations is a formula that estimates the total daily dose of insulin (TDDI) requirement for an adult. For anyone with type 2 diabetes, the calculated TDDI underestimates actual insulin needs.
- There is a tight relationship between the basal insulin dose and the bolus dose as both are calculated using TDDI.

NOTE

1 In the United States or any country that measures blood sugars as mg/dL, the '1800 rule' should be used. Wherever '100' is written, replace with '1800'. For the 72-kg man in the example, 1800/57 = 32. This means that 1 unit of insulin will reduce the blood sugar by 32 mg/dL.

REFERENCES

1. Lebovitz HE. Insulin: potential negative consequences of early routine use of insulin in patients with type 2 diabetes. Diabetes Care. 2011;34(suppl2):S225–S230
2. Bolli GB, Lucidi P, Porcellati F, Fanelli CG. Pivotal role of timely basal insulin replacement after metformin failure in sustaining long-term blood glucose control at a target in type 2 diabetes. Diabetes Care. 2011;34(suppl2);S220–S224
3. Bretzel RG, Nuber U, Landgraf W, et al. Once-daily basal insulin glargine versus thrice-daily prandial insulin lispro in people with type 2 diabetes on oral hypoglycaemic agents (APOLLO): an open randomised controlled trial. Lancet. 2008;371:1073–1084
4. Holman RR, Farmer AJ, Davies MJ, et al. Three-year efficacy of complex insulin regimens in type 2 diabetes. N Engl J Med. 2009;361:1736–1747
5. Inzucchi SE, Bergenstal RM, Buse JB, et al. Management of hypergylcemia in type 2 diabetes: a patient-centred approach. Position statement of the American Diabetes

SUMMARY

- There are two sources of glucose; a continuous 24-hour drip of glucose from the liver, and a sporadic influx through ingestion of food. There are two 'types' of pancreatic insulin secretion: basal to match the hepatic glucose secretion, and bolus to match prandial glucose spikes.
- The guiding principle of exogenous insulin management is to find an insulin regime that best matches a person's physiologic glucose pattern. Thus, it is important to determine each person's physiologic glucose pattern before selecting an insulin regime.
- Many exogenous insulins are available. Traditional insulins are biphasic with both a basal and bolus component. Analogue insulins are monophasic with either a basal or a bolus component.

Association and the European Association of the Study of Diabetes. Diabetes Care. 2012;35:1364–1379

6. O'Connell SM, Cooper MN, Bulsara MK, et al. Reducing rates of severe hypoglycemia in a population-based cohort of children and adolescents with type 1 diabetes over the decade 2000–2009. Diabetes Care. 2011;34:2379–2380

7. Yki-Jarvinen H, Esko N, Eero H, Marja-Riitta T. Clinical benefits and mechanism of a sustained response to intermittent insulin therapy in type 2 diabetes patients with secondary drug failure. Am J Med. 1988;84:185–192

8. McGarry JD, Dobbins RL. Fatty acids, lipotoxicity and insulin secretion. Diabetologia. 1999;42:128–138

9. Marcovecchio ML, Dalton RN, Chiarelli F, Dunger DB. A1c variability as an independent risk factor of microalbuminuria in young people with type 1 diabetes. Diabetes Care. 2011;34:1011–1013

10. Jenkins N, Hallowell N, Farmer AJ, et al. Initiating insulin as part of the treating to target trial in type 2 diabetes (4-T) trial. An interview study of patients' and health professionals' experiences. Diabetes Care. 2010;33:2178–2180

11. Jurinen L, Tiikkainen M, Haddinen AM, et al. Effects of insulin therapy on liver fat content and hepatic insulin sensitivity in patients with type 2 diabetes. Am J Physiol Endocrinol Metab. 2007;292:E829–E835

12. Kotronen A, Westerbacka J, Bergholm R, et al. Liver fat in the metabolic syndrome. J Endocrinol Metab. 2007;92,3490–3497

13. Zachariah S, Sheldon B, Shojaee-Moradie F, et al. Insulin detemir reduces weight gain as a result of reduced food intake in patients with type 1 diabetes. Diabetes Care. 2011;34:1487–1491

14. Giovannucci E, Harlan DM, Archer MC, et al. Diabetes and cancer. ADA consensus report. Diabetes Care. 2010;33:1674–1685

15. ORIGIN Trial Investigators. Basal insulin and cardiovascular and other outcomes in dysglycemia. N Engl J Med. 2012; 367:319–328

16. Gough SCL, Bhargava A, Jain R, et al. Low-volume insulin degludec 200 units/ml once daily improves glycemic control similarly to insulin glargine with low risk of hypoglycaemia in insulin naïve patients with type 2 diabetes. Diabetes Care. 2013;36:2536–2542

17. Fonseca VA. Clinical diabetes: translating research into practice. Saunders Elsevier, Philadelphia, 2006

18. Horvath K, Jeitler K, Berghold A, et al. Long-acting insulin analogues versus NPH insulin (human isophane insulin) for type 2 diabetes mellitus. Cochrane Database Syst Rev. 2007;(2):CD005613

19. Meece J. Needle length and injection technique: size matters. AADE Pract. January 2013:30–31.

20. Blonde L, Merilainen M, Karwe V, Raskin P; TITRATE Study Group. Patient-directed titration for achieving glycaemic goals using a once-daily basal insulin analogue: an assessment of two different fasting plasma glucose targets – the TITRATE study. Diabetes Obes Metab. 2009;11:623–631

21. Famulla S, Hovelmann U, Fischer A, et al. Insulin injection into lipohypertrophic tissue: blunted and more variable insulin absorption and action, and impaired postprandial glucose control. Diabetes Care. 2016;39(9):1486–1492

6

Surgical management of diabetes

METABOLIC/BARIATRIC SURGERY

Originally, bariatric procedures were introduced for weight management. However, with mounting evidence demonstrating sustained reductions in glycaemia and cardiovascular risk, the same procedures are increasingly being used for the management of type 2 diabetes. When performed for this purpose they are called 'metabolic' procedures.[1]

As the gut plays an important role in glucose metabolism, it came as no surprise that bariatric surgery would improve glycaemic control – but the exact mechanisms by which these procedures result in glucose reduction are not well understood.[2]

It should be noted that, despite the evidence, metabolic surgery as a management option for type 2 diabetes has yet to be included within any international diabetes treatment protocols, although in 2016 a joint statement from a group of international experts recommended that metabolic surgery be considered as a treatment option for type 2 diabetes if the BMI is greater than 40 kg/m^2 regardless of glycaemic control and for anyone with a BMI of 35–39.9 kg/m^2 and poorly controlled blood sugars.[1]

The most common metabolic/bariatric procedures performed are Roux-en-Y bypass (RYGB), gastric banding, sleeve gastrectomy and biliopancreatic diversion.[3] All result in weight loss with sustained remission of hyperglycaemia. However, the extent of the weight loss and sustained blood sugar reduction differ between the different approaches. Biliopancreatic diversion provides the best outcomes but has the highest risk of metabolic complications. RYGB achieves better glucose lowering than sleeve gastrectomy, which in turn is better than gastric banding.[1,3]

Roux-en-Y gastric bypass This is the most frequently performed bariatric surgery. As illustrated in Figure 6.1, RYGB begins with the surgical formation of a small stomach pouch. The small intestine is then cut about 75 cm below the stomach. The distal cut end of the small intestine is pulled up and connected to the small stomach pouch (forming one arm of the 'Y') so that ingested food bypasses most of the stomach and part of the small intestine, reducing nutrient absorption. The proximal cut end of the small intestine is then connected to the distal segment of the small intestine (forming the second arm of the 'Y') so that gastric juices, bile and pancreatic exocrine products can enter the duodenum.

Gastric banding Gastric banding (Figure 6.2) reduces stomach volume by placing an adjustable silicone band around the upper part of the stomach to create a smaller 'pre-stomach' pouch. This limits the amount of food that can be consumed at any one time. Post-surgical adjustments to the band to alter stomach volume can be made by injecting fluid into the band through a subcutaneous port.

Sleeve gastrectomy With a sleeve gastrectomy (Figure 6.3), the outer part of the stomach is surgically removed so that it becomes a long narrow tube or 'sleeve'. The reduced gastric volume limits the amount of food that can be consumed at any one time. Unlike gastric banding, the stomach volume cannot be adjusted at a later date.

Biliopancreatic diversion Biliopancreatic diversion (Figure 6.4) is similar to RYGB in that it connects the distal part of the small intestine to the stomach, bypassing the duodenum and jejunum. However, the remnant of the stomach is removed.

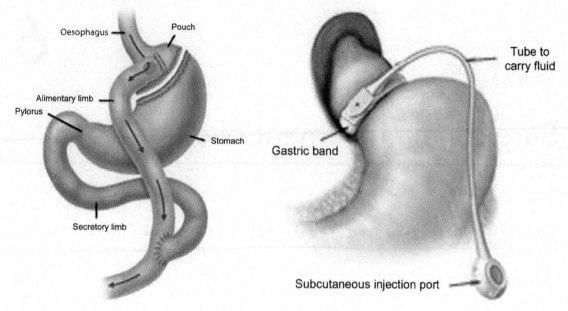

Figure 6.1 Roux-en-Y gastric bypass surgery.

Figure 6.2 Gastric banding.

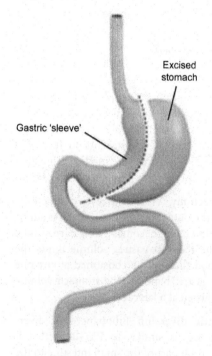

Figure 6.3 Sleeve gastrectomy.

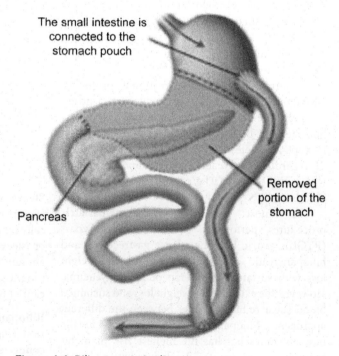

Figure 6.4 Biliopancreatic diversion.

TRANSPLANTATION

Islet cell transplant Islets are harvested from donor pancreases and infused into the recipient's liver. Pancreatic islets include both α-cells, which produce glucagon, and β-cells, which produce insulin. Thus, transplanted islets are able to maintain normal glucose levels as they would in any healthy pancreas. About one-half of islet cell recipients remain completely independent of exogenous insulin a year after islet cell infusion. Even if complete independence from exogenous insulin is not obtained, ongoing glucose control is generally excellent.

Islet cell transplantation is complicated by the need for immunosuppression. This introduces a number of signficant side effects including anaemia, weight loss, hypertension, hyperlipidaemia and nephrotoxity as well as an increased risk of developing cancer. This procedure is still experimental and therefore limited to the management of people with type 1 diabetes who are relatively healthy but have severe hypoglycaemic unawareness that prevents them from holding a job or participating in the usual activities of daily living.

Stem cell transplant Stem cells are the key ingredient for the formation of every tissue in the human body. There are two basic types: embryonic stem cells and adult stem cells. Embryonic stem cells are harvested from the immature cells of an embryo and can be developed into any of the specialist-type cells within a body. In contrast, adult stem cells are harvested from the body after birth (e.g. bone marrow, cord blood) and can only develop into cells particular to the organ or tissue from which they were obtained. For the management of diabetes, stem cells are differentiated into β-cells and transplanted into the recipient.

As with islet cell transplantation, stem cell transplants are limited by the need for long-term immunosuppression. Stem cell transplantation for the management of diabetes is still in the experimental stage and its use limited to those with type 1 diabetes enrolled in studies.

Pancreatic transplant This is a technically difficult surgical procedure and the side effects are significant, so it is typically reserved only for those with type 1 diabetes with serious diabetes complications such as renal failure. A pancreas transplant is generally done in conjunction with a kidney transplant.

SUMMARY

- A number of bariatric procedures are available for the management of diabetes. Roux-en-Y is the most frequently performed.
- There is mounting evidence demonstrating sustained improvement in blood sugars following bariatric surgery. However, metabolic surgery as a management option for type 2 diabetes has yet to be included within any international diabetes treatment protocols.
- Three transplant options exist: islet cell transplant, stem cell transplant and pancreatic transplant. Aside from cost, the biggest barrier to the use of transplants is the need for chronic immunosuppression, increasing the risk for a number of significant medical complications.

REFERENCES

1. Rubino F, Nathan DM, Eckel RH, et al. Delegates of the 2nd Diabetes Surgery Summit. Metabolic surgery in the treatment algorithm for type 2 diabetes: a joint statement by international diabetes organizations. Diabetes Care. 2016:39;861–877
2. Knop FK, Taylor R. Mechanism of metabolic advantages after bariatric surgery. It's all gastrointestinal factors versus it's all food restriction. Diabetes Care. 2013;36(suppl2):S287–S291
3. Buchwald H Avidor Y, Braunwald E, et al. Bariatric surgery: a systematic review and meta-analysis. JAMA. 2004;292:1724–1737

Considerations when approaching diabetes management

This chapter discusses four important concepts that should be considered when approaching diabetes management, especially if the goal is to achieve durable glucose control.

CONSIDER THE PATIENT AS A WHOLE

The demands of diabetes self-management along with medication side effects can positively or negatively affect a patient's sense of well-being, both physically and psychosocially. Thus, when reviewing options for the management of diabetes, it is important to understand and acknowledge each person's medical and psychosocial concerns, including those that are *not* related to their diabetes. Prescribing medications that contribute to weight gain is not going to be well accepted by someone who is struggling to address their weight.

One of the advantages of subscribing to a patient-centred approach, where each person is well informed regarding the pros and cons of each medication and then allowed to participate in the choice of medical management, is the increased likelihood that medical management will address clinical as well as psychological and cultural concerns.

CONSIDER UNDERLYING PATHOLOGY WHEN SELECTING MANAGEMENT OPTIONS

As noted earlier, the American Diabetes Association (ADA) classifies diabetes into four general categories:[1] type 1 diabetes (insulin deficiency secondary to autoimmune destruction of β-cells), type 2 (generally presenting with hyperinsulinaemia with some pancreatic insufficiency but progressing to a more complete insulin deficiency), gestational diabetes and, finally, a 'catch-all' category that includes a long list of rare and not so rare causes of diabetes (e.g. pancreatitis, haemochromatosis, monogenic diabetes, other genetic deficiencies and medications). In a primary care setting, most patients fall into the first two categories; close to 90% are considered type 2, and 10% type 1.[2]

However, when it comes to the clinical management of diabetes, this classification system has three major limitations. First, except for a handful of blood tests (e.g. antibodies, genetic tests) that specifically identify a few types of diabetes, there are no sound objective criteria by which to distinguish one type of diabetes from another.[3,4] This means that identifying or classifying a person's type of diabetes is based on a vague set of clinical parameters such as family history of diabetes, age at disease onset and the presence or absence of the metabolic syndrome. These parameters are not diagnostic but probabilistic, simply providing clues to help categorise a patient.[5] Thus, a child presenting with elevated blood glucose is generally considered to have type 1, while an adult with elevated blood glucose, type 2. Not surprisingly, this imprecise methodology can lead to inaccurate categorisation of patients. With the increasing incidence of obesity in the paediatric population, a child with an elevated blood sugar could have type 2 or type 1 diabetes; likewise, the increased availability of commercial antibody testing has revealed that adults also develop autoimmune diabetes, even in the eighth and ninth decades of life.[6] To further complicate the picture, patients can present with clinical and biochemical features of both type 1 and type 2 diabetes.[7] Currently, it is estimated that up to 20% of adults labelled as having type 2 diabetes do not have type 2 while 5% of those labelled as having type 1 diabetes do not have type 1 – although it is possible that this could be much higher as 20% of those labelled as type 1 did not have positive antibodies at diagnosis.[2,6,8–10]

The second clinical limitation of the ADA classification system is that the categories are defined by what we already know. It is impossible to correctly classify a person with diabetes whose aetiology is yet to be defined. If one were to create a theoretical list of all the possible ways normal glucose metabolism could be disrupted, a large number of causes for hyperglycaemia could be construed: decreased insulin production could be due to autoimmune β-cell destruction, but it could also be due to enzymatic deficiencies in the insulin production pathway, inflammation of the β-cells, or to a deposition-type disease; it could be due to the lack of a cell receptor that turns on a β-cell, due to a liver that does not respond to appropriate feedback around hypoglycaemia or to a problem with any one of the numerous stimulatory hormonal pathways/feedback loops. The presentation of diabetes may have nothing to do with pancreatic dysfunction, but may be due to a defective insulin molecule, mutations of the insulin receptor in the periphery, or defects in the post-receptor signal transduction pathway. The list of possible causes for diabetes is infinite. Many of the pathologies mentioned above are already known and well described, while some are only just beginning to be understood.[6,11,12] Presumably there are many yet to be defined.

Finally, the ADA classification system is limited in its clinical usefulness because of its inability to accurately direct medical management: knowing the type of diabetes a person has does not accurately define their physiologic state. As previously described, regardless of type of diabetes, each person has a unique set of pathologies contributing to their diabetes. Furthermore, the extent to which different pathologies contribute to the expression of the disease can change over time. Early on in type 2 diabetes an individual is hyperinsulinaemic with peripheral insulin resistance, but with disease progression they may become increasingly insulin-deficient. Despite this understanding, however, providers continue to base management choices on the type of diabetes a person has. For those labelled as having type 2 diabetes, advice for lifestyle modification is offered initially, followed by the introduction of oral medications in a stepwise fashion as the disease progresses. Which oral hypoglycaemic is used first, and the order in which subsequent medications are added, is largely determined by guidelines, physician preference, patient tolerance and trial and error.[13] The choice has little to do with targeting specific deficiencies in the patient's glucose metabolic pathway.

As outlined in the previous chapter, multiple classes of treatment agents are now available, each class targeting a specific aspect of the glucose metabolic pathway. Metformin reduces hepatic gluconeogenesis, sulfonylureas and meglitinides increase endogenous insulin secretion, thiazolidinediones increase peripheral insulin sensitivity and α-glucosidase inhibitors decrease glucose absorption in the gut. Exogenous insulin obviously increases insulin supply. More recently, exogenous incretins that modulate gut hormones have become available. With such diversity in available treatments, we now have the ability to tailor medical management to specific pathologies. Thus, understanding which pathologies are contributing to a person's hyperglycaemia, rather than what type of diabetes they have, is paramount when decisions are being made about medical management.[14]

However, clinical deficiencies aside, there are important reasons as to why a person's type of diabetes should be established. These include the following:

- Certain types of diabetes do dictate specific management choices: e.g. the GCK variant of monogenic diabetes requires no treatment; the HNF-1α and HNF-4α variants of monogenic diabetes are preferentially managed with sulfonylureas.
- For the types of diabetes with strong genetic components (e.g. haemochromatosis, monogenic diabetes), making a correct diagnosis could lead to timely genetic testing of family members, resulting in earlier and better tailoring of management for others.

- It is likely that management options for different types of diabetes will continue to improve and multiply. Making an accurate diagnosis would enable timely identification of those who would benefit from these new advances.
- Healthcare systems (private or public) continue to base funding decisions for selected management options on types of diabetes, e.g. insulin pumps for those with type 1 diabetes. Until healthcare systems change to basing decisions on pathological states (e.g. insulin deficiency), establishing each individual's type of diabetes will ensure access to entitled management options.

CONSIDER THE DURABILITY OF MANAGEMENT

Two different approaches to the treatment of diabetes are possible: the traditional 'guideline' approach and the 'pathophysiologic' approach.[15]

The guideline approach is widely accepted and promoted as current best practice within most clinical settings internationally – especially for the management of type 2 diabetes. This approach promotes the sequential addition of management options (lifestyle and medical) to achieve an HbA_{1c} target. Critics have labelled this the 'treat to failure' approach, as escalation of medical management only occurs when a patient is not reaching their glycaemic target. Thus, as disease progression is a given, all patients will cycle in and out of good glycaemic control as they repeatedly fail each newly added medication.[16]

In contrast, the 'pathophysiologic' approach advocates the initiation of a combination of therapies at the onset of disease with the goal of producing a durable reduction in HbA_{1c}. Medications are selected based on the need to target the specific pathophysiologic disturbances contributing to a person's hyperglycaemia.[17] Thus, if three underlying pathologies are seen to be contributing to the person's diabetes, then three agents, each targeting one of the pathologies, should be selected. Proponents of this approach also emphasise the need to be "cognizant of the ABCDE[1] of diabetes management":[15] i.e. the choice of medication should not just be based on its glucose-lowering efficacy and durability, but also on its ability to manage weight, blood pressure, lipids and cardiovascular risk.

DETERMINE THE PATIENT'S TYPE OF DIABETES AND UNDERLYING PATHOLOGIES

Ideally, determining a patient's type of diabetes should be dependent on a set of objective data. However, we do not have a complete set of diagnostic tests that can accurately distinguish all types of diabetes. This often makes confirmation of type of diabetes a significant challenge.[3,4] For a few, such as type 1 and monogenic diabetes, confirmation can be made with blood tests. For most types, however, establishing the type and determining the underlying pathologies must be garnered from the patient's medical history, family history and clinical presentation. Blood sugar checks, insulin doses and laboratory tests are then used to strengthen or weaken clinical suspicions.

Thus, determining a person's diagnosis and underlying physiology depends on honing one's history-taking skills and on having a good understanding of the characteristics of each type of diabetes and their respective underlying pathologies, as well as the family history and clinical presentations associated with each.

It is my belief that every provider meeting a person with diabetes for the first time should make no conclusions about that patient's type of diabetes and contributing pathologies until a complete medical history and full clinical exam has been completed. A complete medical history necessarily includes the patient's medical history at the time of diagnosis, a history of the course and management of the diabetes since diagnosis and the patient's family medical history.

Management of the more uncommon types of diabetes is specialist level care and beyond the scope of this manual. However, all providers managing patients with diabetes should be able to recognise clinical presentations suggestive of atypical diabetes. The tables below provide a comprehensive list of questions to be included during a complete history taking – remembering, of course, that the answers given by the person are not diagnostic, but simply providing a set of clues that aid clinical decision-making.

Table 7.1 Patient history

Question	Clinical significance
How were you diagnosed with diabetes? Was the diagnosis made from a screening test or had you presented with a clinical complaint?	Receiving the diagnosis of diabetes following a screening test is more suggestive of type 2 diabetes, less suggestive of primary pancreatic failure.
Were you losing weight or thirsty, or did you have urinary frequency at diagnosis?	Weight loss, urinary frequency and thirst suggest significant pancreatic failure.
How old were you at diagnosis?	While type 1 and type 2 diabetes can present at any age, the probability that a child/young adult does not have type 2 is still higher. The more common types of monogenic diabetes present in young adulthood or early thirties.
What is your ethnicity?	Different ethnicities carry higher risks for certain types of diabetes. The genetics behind this is still poorly understood, but a growing area of interest.
How much did you weigh at time of diagnosis?	Lack of obesity suggests lack of insulin resistance.
Were you physically active at the time of diagnosis? Were you playing any sports? If so, at what level were you playing?	A new diagnosis of diabetes in a 30 year old who played sport throughout their school years is less likely to have insulin resistance contributing to disease onset.
Were you acutely unwell at diagnosis? Were you hospitalised?	Hospitalisation secondary to diabetes at diagnosis implies ketosis or ketoacidosis (late diagnosis of type 2 diabetes or type 1 diabetes).
Do you know if you had ketones at the time of diagnosis?	Ketones at presentation are suggestive of significant pancreatic failure.
When you first got diabetes, how were you told to manage it? Were you given any medications? If so, which medications? Did you tolerate the medications or have any problems with the medications?	A rapid progression from oral medications onto insulin is suggestive of insulin deficiency secondary to pancreatic insufficiency – or a rapid progression of pancreatic failure (think autoimmunity, pancreatitis or pancreatic cancer).
Are you on insulin? How much? How soon after diagnosis were you put on the insulin?	Small doses of insulin support a likelihood of insulin sensitivity; large doses support a likelihood of insulin resistance.
Have you ever been on a sulfonylurea? Did you ever have a hypoglycaemic episode when you were taking a sulfonylurea?	Having a hypoglycaemic event on a sulfonylurea suggests insulin sensitivity; i.e. type 2 diabetes is less likely.
Have you ever been on a glitizone? Did adding a glitizone improve your blood sugars?	No improvement in blood sugars when on a glitizone suggests a lack of peripheral insulin resistance.

Table 7.2 Past medical history

Question	Clinical significance
Do you drink alcohol? How much?	1–3% of heavy alcohol drinkers (defined as consuming 4–5 drinks of alcohol per day) will develop acute pancreatitis over a span of 10–20 years.[18]
Do you smoke? How much?	Smoking is associated with insulin resistance and the development of type 2 diabetes.[19]
Do you have a history of gestational diabetes? If yes, in what trimester was the diagnosis of diabetes made? Do you have a history of delivering large or small babies?	Placental hormones in the final trimester of pregnancy significantly increase insulin resistance. Thus, the development of diabetes in the third trimester signifies a pancreas incapable of rising to the challenge of higher insulin needs. Insulin resistance does not increase in the first and second trimesters of pregnancy. Thus, the development of diabetes within the first two trimesters suggests primary pancreatic dysfunction.
Have you ever been ill or had surgery (e.g. pancreatectomy, cholecystectomy)?	Gallstones can remain in the common bile duct following a cholecystectomy, increasing the risk of developing pancreatitis.
Do you have a history of other autoimmune diseases (e.g. coeliac disease, autoimmune thyroid disease, rheumatoid arthritis, vitiligo)?	Having an autoimmune disease increases the likelihood of autoimmune diabetes.
Do you have any skin rashes (e.g. psoriatic-like scaley patches, dermatitis herpetiformis, nail dystrophies, acanthosis nigricans)?	Acanthosis nigricans is associated with insulin resistance. Skin rashes can indicate the presence of autoimmunity.
Do you have any problems with hearing? Muscle weakness? Developmental delay?	There are a number of rare genetic disorders with syndromic presentations that include elevated blood sugars/diabetes.
Have you ever been told that you have a problem with your liver? Or have elevated liver enzymes?	Raised liver enzymes may signify fatty liver disease, which is associated with insulin resistance and the development of type 2 diabetes.
Do you have sleep apnoea?	Sleep apnoea contributes to the development of insulin resistance.[20]

Table 7.3 Family history

Question	Clinical significance
Who else has diabetes in your family?	This should be a comprehensive review of at least three generations. The presence of diabetes in multiple family members in multiple generations is suggestive of a genetic cause of diabetes.
For each family member with diabetes: • What type of diabetes do they have? • How old were they when they were diagnosed? • Were they obese or thin at the time of their diagnosis? • Were they physically active at the time of diagnosis? • Are they on pills or on insulin? ▪ If on insulin, how soon after diagnosis were they put on insulin? ▪ Do you know what doses of insulin they are on? ▪ Do they take insulin at meal times? • Were any of them losing weight at time of diagnosis? • Do any of them have hypertension, high cholesterol?	A red flag for monogenic diabetes is a family with many members with diabetes, some carrying the diagnosis of type 1 and some carrying the diagnosis of type 2. See above for the clinical significance of these questions.
Is there any family history of autoimmune/ genetic diseases?	For example: haemochromatosis, coeliac disease, rheumatoid arthritis, ankylosing spondylitis, thyroid, psoriasis, etc.

Table 7.4 Clinical presentation of the patient

Feature	Clinical significance
Weight, body mass index, waist circumference	Central obesity is an indication of insulin resistance, raising the likelihood of type 2 diabetes – but it does not rule out other types.
Blood pressure	The presence of hypertension (along with central obesity) raises the likelihood of metabolic syndrome/type 2 diabetes.
Cholesterol profile	High triglycerides + high LDL is suggestive of type 2 diabetes/metabolic syndrome. High HDL (> 1.1 mmol/L or 42.5 mg/dL) suggests lack of metabolic syndrome; less likely to be type 2 diabetes.
Enlarged liver, elevated liver function tests Ultrasound with fatty infiltration of the liver	The presence of elevated liver function tests raises the possibility of fatty liver. The presence of a fatty liver increases the likelihood of insulin resistance/type 2 diabetes.

Table 7.5 Useful blood tests

Blood test	Clinical significance
Oral glucose tolerance test (OGTT) The test includes a fasting blood glucose (FBG) and a blood glucose check 1 and/or 2 hours following a 75-g glucose challenge.	The OGTT reflects the pathophysiology behind diabetes better than any other glycaemic parameter.[21] Each result provides different information about a person's underlying physiologic state. An abnormal FBG demonstrates hepatic insulin resistance, β-cell dysfunction[22-24] and reduced β-cell mass.[25] An abnormal post-glucose challenge reflects increased peripheral insulin resistance with near-normal hepatic insulin sensitivity and progressive loss of β-cell function.[22,23,25]
Liver function tests (LFTs)	LFTs should always be checked at diagnosis of diabetes. If elevated, further work-up to determine the aetiology should be completed. A number of diseases that cause elevated LFTs are associated with the development of hyperglycaemia. These include: • Haemochromatosis. With a prevalence of 1 in 200, haemochromatosis continues to be under-recognised as a cause of preventable diabetes.[26] • Fatty liver (non-alcoholic steatohepatitis). • Diseases of the liver, including all viral hepatitides, α-1 antitrypsin disease.
Fasting C-peptide and FBG The current gold standard for assessment of β-cell function and insulin sensitivity is the hyperinsulinaemic–euglycaemic clamp.[27,28] However, this method is labour-intensive, costly and impractical for clinical application. Simpler surrogate indices, such as the fasting C-peptide concentration, can be used.[12,27-32] While C-peptide measurement has been criticised for its lack of reproducibility, numerous studies have established its clinical usefulness with regard to characterisation of insulin production and peripheral insulin resistance.[12,28,31-34]	Of note, the C-peptide result can only be interpreted if a simultaneous FBG result is available. • A fasting C-peptide concentration within normal range reflects normal β-cell function only if the FBG is in normal range. • A fasting C-peptide concentration within normal range with an elevated FBG indicates pancreatic insufficiency. • As greater insulin secretion is necessary to produce an equivalent level of glycaemia in the face of greater insulin resistance, a fasting C-peptide concentration higher than normal with an FBG of 6 mmol/L (110 mg/dL) suggests sufficient pancreatic function, but relative insulin resistance. • A fasting C-peptide concentration that is higher than normal accompanied by an FBG of 20 mmol/L (360 mg/dL) characterises a person with significant peripheral insulin resistance and relative pancreatic deficiency.
Antibodies Of note, checking antibodies is limited in late disease as they fade over time.	Antibody tests for establishing the diagnosis of type 1 diabetes include: • Glutamic acid decarboxylase antibody (GAD) • Islet cell antibody (ICA) • Insulin auto-antibody (IAA) • Zinc transporter auto-antibody (ZNT8)
Genetic testing	If a genetic cause for diabetes is suspected, specialist advice should be sought with regard to appropriate tests.

SUMMARY

- When selecting options for the management of diabetes, it is important to understand and acknowledge each person's medical and psychosocial concerns, including those unrelated to their diabetes.
- The ADA classification system for diabetes is limited in its clinical usefulness as
  - it relies on putative aetiologies underlying the different types of diabetes,
  - the categories are defined by what we already know; there is no place for a person with diabetes whose aetiology is yet to be defined,
  - it does not accurately reflect a person's physiologic state, a necessary understanding for tailoring medical management.
- The current 'guideline approach' to diabetes management advocates for the sequential addition of medications, with the goal of achieving a target HbA_{1c}. This invariably results in a person's cycling in and out of good diabetes control. In contrast, the 'pathophysiologic approach' to diabetes management uses combination therapy at the onset of disease with the goal of producing a durable reduction in HbA_{1c}.
- We do not have a set of diagnostic tests that can accurately distinguish all types of diabetes. Clues for establishing type of diabetes and determining underlying pathologies must often be garnered from a patient's medical history, family history and clinical presentation. Blood sugar checks, insulin doses and laboratory tests can be used to strengthen or weaken clinical suspicions.
- All providers managing patients with diabetes should be able to recognise clinical presentations suggestive of atypical diabetes.

NOTE

1 A, age; B, body weight; C, complications (micro-vascular and macrovascular); D, duration of diabetes; E, life expectancy; E, expense.

REFERENCES

1. American Diabetes Association. Classification and diagnosis of diabetes: standards of medical care in diabetes – 2019. Diabetes Care. 2019;42(suppl1):S13–S28
2. Engelgau MM, Narayan KMV, Herman WH. Screening for type 2 diabetes. Diabetes Care. 2000;23:1563–1580
3. Silverstein J, Klingensmith G, Copeland K, et al. Care of children and adolescents with type 1 diabetes: a statement of the American Diabetes Association. Diabetes Care. 2005;28:186–212
4. Ehtisham S, Barrett TG. The emergence of type 2 diabetes in childhood. Ann Clin Biochem. 2004;41:10–16
5. Harron KL, Feltbower RG, McKinney PA, et al. Rising rates of all types of diabetes in South Asian and non-South Asian children and young people aged 0–29 years in West Yorkshire, UK, 1991–2006. Diabetes Care. 2011;34:652–654
6. American Diabetes Association. Type 2 diabetes in children and adolescents. Diabetes Care. 2000;23:381–389
7. Copeland KC, Becker D, Gottshalk M, Hale D. Type 2 diabetes in children and adolescents: risk factors, diagnosis and treatment. Clin Diabetes. 2005;23:181–185
8. Juneja R, Hirsch IB, Naik RG, et al. Islet cell antibodies and GAD antibodies, but not clinical phenotype help identify type 1½ diabetes in patients presenting with type 2 diabetes. Metabolism. 2001;50:1008–1013
9. Nesmith JD. Type 2 diabetes in children and adolescents. Pediatr Rev. 2001;22:147–152
10. Turner R, Stratton I, Horton V, et al. UKPDS 25: autoantibodies to islet-cell cytoplasm and glutamic acid decarboxylase for prediction of insulin requirement in type 2 diabetes. Lancet. 1997;350:1288–1293
11. Winter WE, Nakamura M, House DV. Monogenic diabetes mellitus in youth. The MODY syndromes. Endocrinol Metab Clin North Am. 1999;28:765–785
12. Bergman RN, Watanabe R, Rebrin K, et al. Toward an integrated

phenotype in pre-NIDDM. Diabet Med. 1996:13(suppl6):S67–S77

13. Tan MH, Baksi A, Kuahulec B, et al. Comparison of pioglitizone and gliclazide in sustaining glycemic control over 2 years in patients with type 2 diabetes. Diabetes Care. 2005;28(3):544–550

14. American Diabetes Association. Diagnosis and classification of diabetes mellitus. Diabetes Care. 2012;35(suppl1):S64–S71

15. DeFronzo RA, Eldor R, Abdul-Ghani M. Pathophysiologic approach to therapy in patients with newly diagnosed type 2 diabetes. Diabetes Care. 2013;36:S127–S138

16. Schernthaner G, Barnett AH, Betteridge DJ, et al. Is the ADA/EASD algorithm for the management of type 2 diabetes (January 2009) based on evidence or opinion? A critical analysis. Diabetologia. 2010;53:1258–1269

17. Defronzo RA. Banting Lecture. From the triumvirate to the ominous octet: a new paradigm for the treatment of type 2 diabetes mellitus. Diabetes. 2009;58:773–795

18. Sadr AO, Orsini N, Andren-Sandberg A, et al. Effect of type of alcoholic beverage in causing acute pancreatitis. Br J Surg. 2011;98:1609–1616

19. Willi C, Bodenmann P, Ghali WA, et al. Active smoking and the risk of type 2 diabetes: a systematic review and meta-analysis. JAMA. 2007;298:2654–2664

20. Ip MSM, Lam B, Ng MMT, et al. Obstructive sleep apnea is independently associated with insulin resistance. Am J Respir Crit Care Med. 2002;165:670–676

21. Bonora E, Tuomilehto J. The pros and cons of diagnosing diabetes with A1c. Diabetes Care. 2011;34(suppl2):S184–S190

22. Nathan DM, Davidson MB, DeFronzo RA, et al. Impaired fasting glucose and impaired glucose tolerance: implications for care. Diabetes Care. 2007;30:753–759

23. Abdul-Ghani MA, Tripathy D, DeFronzo RA. Contributions of β-cell dysfunction and insulin resistance to the pathogenesis of impaired glucose tolerance and impaired fasting glucose. Diabetes Care. 2006;29:1130–1139

24. Faerch K, Vaag A, Holst JJ, et al. Natural history of insulin sensitivity and insulin secretion in the progression from normal glucose tolerance to impaired fasting glycemia and impaired glucose tolerance: the Inter99 study. Diabetes Care. 2009;32:439–444

25. Faerch K, Borch-Johnsen K, Holst JJ, Vaag A. Pathophysiology and aetiology of impaired fasting glycaemia and impaired glucose tolerance: does it matter for prevention treatment of type 2 diabetes? Diabetologia. 2009;52:1714–1723

26. Borgaonkar MR. Hemochromatosis. More common that you think. Can Fam Physician. 2003;49:36–43

27. Matsuda M. Insulin sensitivity indices obtained from oral glucose tolerance testing. Comparison with the euglycemic insulin clamp. Diabetes Care. 1999;22:1462–1470

28. Tripathy D, Almgren P, Tuomi T, Groop L. Contribution of insulin-stimulated glucose uptake and basal hepatic insulin sensitivity to surrogate measures of insulin sensitivity. Diabetes Care. 2004;27:2204–2210

29. The Diabetes Control and Complications Trial Research Group. The effect of intensive treatment of diabetes on the development and progression of long-term complication in insulin-dependent diabetes mellitus. N Engl J Med. 1993;329:977–986

30. Bloomgarden ZT. Thiazolidinediones. Diabetes Care. 2005;28:488–493

31. Laakso M. How good a marker is insulin level for insulin resistance? Am J Epidemiol. 1993;137:959–965

32. Sluter WJ, Erkelens DW, Reitsma WD, et al. Glucose tolerance and insulin release, a mathematical approach. I. Assay of the beta-cell response after oral glucose loading. Diabetes. 1976;25:241–244

33. Sluter WJ, Erkelens DW, Terpstra P, et al. Glucose tolerance and insulin release, a mathematical approach. II. Approximation of the peripheral insulin resistance after oral glucose loading. Diabetes. 1976;25:245–249

34. Matthews DR, Hosker JP, Rudenski AS, et al. Homeostasis model assessment: insulin resistance and beta-cell function from fasting plasma glucose and insulin concentrations in man. Diabetologia. 1985;28:412–419

8

Glycaemic management

MEDICAL MANAGEMENT OF GLYCAEMIA

For both providers and patients, managing diabetes is synonymous with managing blood sugars. However, it is important to remember that the primary reason for managing diabetes is to lower a person's cardiovascular risk. The accepted measure of cardiovascular risk related to diabetes is HbA_{1c}, with the understanding that a reduction of 11 mmol/mol (1%) in HbA_{1c} will result in a "37% decrease in risk for microvascular complications and a 21% decrease in the risk of any end point of death related to diabetes."[1]

HbA_{1c} is also, of course, a measure of a person's average blood sugars over the past 3 months – a fact that we often share with our patients. However, I would argue that, in terms of achieving long-term behavioural changes, it is more important for patients to understand the association between their HbA_{1c} and their cardiovascular risk/long-term health rather than what their average blood sugar is. Indeed, when I ask patients what their understanding of normal blood sugar is in someone without diabetes, I rarely if ever get the correct answer. So being told their average blood sugar is likely going to be fairly meaningless. Instructions on how to explain HbA_{1c} and its associated cardiovascular risk can be found in Chapter 10, Cardiovascular Risk Management.

It is also important that patients understand what the expected improvement in HbA_{1c} is with each management choice. A general rule of thumb is that the first oral medication will reduce HbA_{1c} by 11 mmol/mol (1%), possibly 15 mmol/mol (1.5%).[2,3] This reduction in HbA_{1c} occurs regardless of the class of medication selected. How significant

the improvement is depends on a number of factors, including how early in the disease process the medication is introduced, how well the patient engages in lifestyle changes and how high the HbA_{1c} is at the time the oral medication is initiated. The higher the HbA_{1c}, the greater the improvement one can expect.

For each additional medication one can expect a further HbA_{1c} reduction of 5 mmol/mol (half a percentage point). Thus, for a person with an HbA_{1c} of 86 mmol/mol (10%), the first medication will bring their HbA_{1c} to around 75 mmol/mol (9%); adding a second oral medication will bring the HbA_{1c} down to around 70 mmol/mol (8.5%); while a third oral medication would get the HbA_{1c} down to 65 mmol/mol (8.1%). Clearly, when a patient presents with a high HbA_{1c}, insulin as a management option will need to be discussed, if not initiated, immediately. The American Diabetes Association recommends introducing insulin if the HbA_{1c} is 75 mmol/mol (9%),[4] while the American Association of Clinical Endocrinologists recommends initiating insulin when the HbA_{1c} is 64 mmol/mol (8%).[5]

Glucose variability also contributes to cardiovascular risk.[6] Thus, a person with an HbA_{1c} of 64 mmol/mol (8%) with widely swinging sugars is at a higher cardiovascular risk than a person with the same HbA_{1c} and little variability in their blood sugars. With the advent and increasing popularity of continuous glucose monitoring, there has been a renewed interest in monitoring for glucose variability.[7]

INDIVIDUALISATION OF HBA_{1c} TARGET

As lower HbA_{1c} correlates with lower cardiovascular risk, the assumption guiding diabetes management has been 'lower is better'. Indeed, the history of the development of medications and insulins reflects the drive to produce products that can more effectively lower HbA_{1c} without increasing the risk of hypoglycaemia. In 2011 two studies, the ACCORD and the ADVANCE, set out to corroborate this assumption.[8,9] Each took a large population of adults with diabetes and attempted to drive HbA_{1c} to below 47 mmol/mol (6.5%). For some participants these attempts to tighten HbA_{1c} resulted in increased cardiovascular events and all-cause mortality. Retrospective analysis found these participants to be elderly individuals with multiple chronic conditions, on multiple medications and with high cardiovascular risk scores. It is still not entirely clear why this group did particularly poorly, but the ensuing consensus has been that lower is not necessarily better, that patients should not be held to identical HbA_{1c} targets and that glycaemic goals should be individualised.[10,11]

To date, no clear guidelines have been provided as to what factors should influence decisions around individualisation of HbA_{1c} targets. Based on the findings from the ACCORD and ADVANCE trials, recommendations suggest considering less stringent control in those with many years of diabetes, high cardiovascular risk, multiple chronic conditions with multiple medications, the use of insulin, the presence of hypoglycaemic unawareness and short life expectancy.[2]

The frequency of checking HbA_{1c} should also be individualised. For patients with unstable, uncontrolled diabetes or with recent changes in medical management, HbA_{1c} should be tested every 3 months. For those whose HbA_{1c} is at target and at low risk for hypoglycaemia, twice-yearly checks are considered reasonable.[12]

SELF-MONITORING OF BLOOD SUGARS

Routine self-monitoring of blood sugars should only be done if the resultant blood glucose value is going to contribute to management decision-making. This means that not all people with diabetes need to check their blood sugars. In fact, regular self-monitoring of blood glucose in people with type 2 diabetes who are not on insulin has been shown to provide limited clinical benefit.[13] Obviously, access to glucose monitoring for those at risk for hypoglycaemia is recommended.

This means that:

- A person managing their diabetes with lifestyle changes and/or oral medications at low risk for causing hypoglycaemia should not be instructed to check their blood sugar every day.
- A person on oral medications that puts them at risk for hypoglycaemia or on a stable dose of basal insulin should not be instructed to check their blood sugar every day. However, access and instruction on the use of a blood glucose meter is necessary for the management of hypoglycaemia. Checking blood sugars is also necessary when a decision around medical management is wanting to be made, e.g. when HbA_{1c} is not at target.
- For a person using a basal insulin, periodic blood sugar checks to monitor for disease progression, along with instructions on how to titrate insulin dosing, can assist with durable diabetes control.
- A person on a flexible or semi-flexible insulin regime should, at a minimum, be checking blood sugars prior to each meal to determine appropriate insulin doses for that meal.
- It is questionable whether a person using a fixed basal–bolus insulin regime or insulin mix should check blood sugars prior to meals as the blood glucose is not being used to adjust insulin doses. However, access and instruction on the use of a blood glucose meter is necessary for the management of hypoglycaemia.
- A person on insulin and/or a sulfonylurea who is unwell should check blood sugars regularly to monitor for excessively high or low blood sugars.

Hand-held blood glucose meters are the most common way for people to monitor their blood sugars (Figure 8.1). Using blood obtained from a fingerprick, the result displayed on the meter screen represents the person's blood sugar at that point in time. The meter provides no information that allows the user to predict whether the blood sugars are trending up or down.

Multiple blood glucose meters are available, each with its own features. Most meters run on batteries, some are rechargeable. Older meters require calibration before they can be used. Most meters these days will store multiple blood sugar results which can later be downloaded for ease of review; some

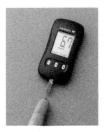

Figure 8.1 Hand-held blood glucose meter.

are Bluetooth or plug into mobile phones, with any number of apps to facilitate analysis of blood sugars. Some meters connect via Bluetooth to insulin pumps; others can be used to check both ketones and blood sugars. 'Talking' meters for the visually impaired are also available. Of note, blood glucose and ketone strips are specific for each meter. Finally, an 0800 number can be found on the back of each meter should assistance be needed or for ordering equipment (e.g. batteries, cords and programs for downloading).

A continuous glucose monitoring (CGM) system differs from a hand-held blood glucose meter in that a subcutaneous glucose sensor is worn 24 hours a day. As the sensor is not in a blood vessel, but positioned interstitially, the glucose value is a surrogate blood glucose value. However, the results from the interstitial glucose checks have been shown to correlate well with plasma glucose.[13] The sensor checks sugars at frequent and regular intervals (approximately every 5 minutes). This information is then communicated to a receiver for the user to review. Depending on the CGM model, the receiver may be a hand-held device, a mobile phone, a watch or an insulin pump. Because the sugars are being checked continually, the information is relayed as a 24-hour tracing, providing information about the blood sugar at any point in time as well as information on whether the sugars are trending up or down.

Two different types of CGM systems are available. A real-time CGM system, as described above, continuously feeds glucose information to the receiver regardless of whether the user is looking at the receiver. The receiver comes equipped with alarms that can alert the wearer to rapid rises or drops in their blood sugars. The second type of CGM available – more accurately called a continuous blood glucose meter – does not continually feed information to the receiver in real time. While the sensor is checking the glucose at regular

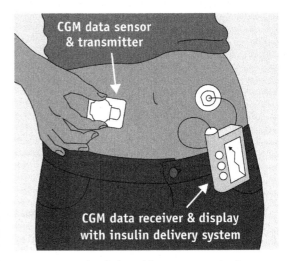

Figure 8.2 Hybrid closed-loop system. A glucose sensor relays real-time information to the insulin pump, which automatically adjusts insulin delivery to maintain blood sugars within target range.

intervals, the information is only relayed to the receiver when the wearer actively 'scans' the glucose sensor.

Modern, sophisticated insulin pumps receiving blood glucose information from a sensor are now capable of automatically suspending insulin delivery or adjusting insulin delivery based on glucose sensor readings. These are often referred to as 'closed-loop systems' (Figure 8.2).

BLOOD GLUCOSE MANAGEMENT

Diabetes management decisions require a review of both the HbA_{1c} and the blood sugars. Each of these provides very different information from the other, and both pieces of information are necessary if correct management decisions are to be made. This is true regardless of what management regime a person is on.

The HbA_{1c} tells us *whether* the person's management regime needs to be changed; it does not provide any information on *what* changes need to be made; i.e. if HbA_{1c} is the only information available, no decisions around management should be made. This includes making the decision not to change a current management regime when a person's HbA_{1c} is at target and the patient is on a sulfonylurea or insulin, as they may be having hypoglycaemic episodes.

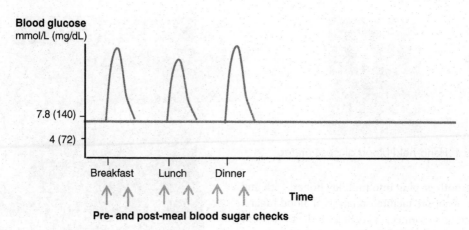

Figure 8.3 The physiologic glucose pattern of a person with poorly controlled mealtime sugars.

Blood sugar checks tell us *what* needs to be changed. Pre- and post-meal blood glucose checks provide very specific information about a person's physiologic glucose pattern, thereby directing exactly what changes need to be made to the management regime. A blood glucose check first thing in the morning reflects how well oral medications and/or basal insulin (endogenous or exogenous) are matching hepatic glucose production, while post-meal blood glucose checks reflect how well endogenous pancreatic function is meeting the increased insulin needs with the influx of carbohydrates, how well exogenous insulin dosing is matching the influx of carbohydrates with ingestion, or how well exogenous gut hormone preparations are resulting in appropriate endogenous insulin production. Figure 8.3 is a schematic of pre- and post-meal blood sugars demonstrating a clear need for improved mealtime management.

One final important reason for reviewing HbA_{1c} and blood sugars together is to ensure that the HbA_{1c} aligns with the person's blood sugars. An HbA_{1c} result not only reflects the person's blood sugars but is also dependent on the size and quantity (amongst other parameters) of haemoglobin. Anaemia and haemoglobinopathies are two common reasons why an HbA_{1c} may not be a true reflection of the person's blood sugars.

For those using a hand-held blood glucose meter, 2 or 3 days of pre- and post-meal blood sugars provides ample information for any decision-making around management changes.

Unfortunately, a person does not usually present for a diabetes check with a nice schematic graph of blood sugars as presented in Figure 8.3. Rather, you are likely to end up with a page full of numbers from a computer download, or the patient will bring a page of documented sugars such as those written below:

mmol/L (mg/dL)	Before breakfast	After breakfast	Before lunch	After lunch	Before dinner	After dinner
Monday	6.7 (122)	17.3 (312)	9.1 (164)	20 (360)	9 (162)	24.4 (440)
Tuesday	8.9 (160)	23.3 (420)	12.7 (228)	19.1 (344)	10.2 (184)	21.6 (388)
Wednesday	8.1 (146)	19.6 (352)	10.1 (182)	18.3 (330)	8.8 (158)	20.3 (366)

If you are struggling to make sense out of the numbers, translate them into a graph. In fact, Figure 8.3 is a schematic depiction of the above blood sugars. Representing the numbers as a schematic facilitates pattern recognition, clarifies interpretation and makes it obvious as to what management options one should be considering to resolve the patients high HbA$_{1c}$.

To create a graph from the page of numbers, take a highlighting pen and highlight all the pre-meal blood sugars, so that the page of numbers now looks like the chart below:

mmol/L (mg/dL)	Before breakfast	After breakfast	Before lunch	After lunch	Before dinner	After dinner
Monday	6.7 (122)	17.3 (312)	9.1 (164)	20 (360)	9 (162)	24.4 (440)
Tuesday	8.9 (160)	23.3 (420)	12.7 (228)	19.1 (344)	10.2 (184)	21.6 (388)
Wednesday	8.1 (146)	19.6 (352)	10.1 (182)	18.3 (330)	8.8 (158)	20.3 (366)

Now the patterns become more obvious. It is clear that this person is

- consistently waking with an average blood sugar of around 8 mmol/L (144 mg/dL), and
- consistently spiking after every meal.

Superimposing the schematic of a normal physiologic glucose pattern onto the schematic representation of the patient's blood sugars (Figure 8.4) can also be very helpful when trying to get a patient to understand what changes need to be made to their management.

Subsequent management decisions are then based on attempting to line up the patient's blood glucose pattern with the normal physiologic glucose pattern; e.g. if the patient whose blood sugars are represented in Figure 8.4 is on insulin, the basal insulin should be increased and mealtime insulin doses increased (or carbohydrate intake decreased).

Similarly, a second set of blood sugars may look like this:

mmol/L (mg/dL)	Before breakfast	After breakfast	Before lunch	After lunch	Before dinner	After dinner
Monday	15.9 (286)	14.9 (268)	15.6 (280)	17.8 (320)	16.1 (290)	15.1 (272)
Tuesday	14.4 (260)	18.9 (340)	15.1 (272)	13.4 (242)	15.3 (276)	19.3 (348)
Wednesday	17.4 (314)	16.2 (292)	13 (234)	13.6 (244)	17.1 (308)	15.9 (286)

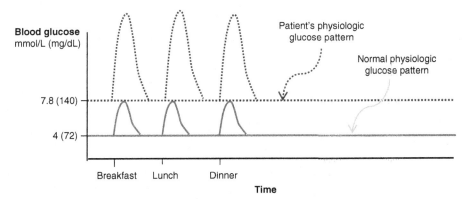

Figure 8.4 The physiologic glucose pattern of a person with poorly controlled fasting and mealtime sugars.

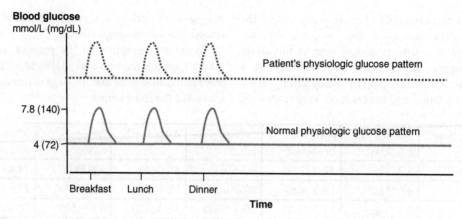

Figure 8.5 The physiologic glucose pattern of a person with poorly controlled fasting sugars.

Highlighting all the pre-meal blood sugars will produce the following chart:

mmol/L (mg/dL)	Before breakfast	After breakfast	Before lunch	After lunch	Before dinner	After dinner
Monday	15.9 (286)	14.9 (268)	15.6 (280)	17.8 (320)	16.1 (290)	15.1 (272)
Tuesday	14.4 (260)	18.9 (340)	15.1 (272)	13.4 (242)	15.3 (276)	19.3 (348)
Wednesday	17.4 (314)	16.2 (292)	13 (234)	13.6 (244)	17.1 (308)	15.9 (286)

Clearly, this person only has a problem with their fasting blood sugars as there are no mealtime spikes. This is depicted schematically in Figure 8.5. Choices of management for this patient would include escalation of oral medications, starting a basal insulin or, if they are already on a basal insulin, increasing the dose.

How to read and interpret blood sugars is a very important skill to master. It is also an extremely important skill to teach to patients. This is discussed further in Chapter 12, Empowering the Patient for Lifelong Self-Management.

The principles behind interpreting blood sugars from a CGM system are identical; in fact, downloaded blood sugar information is automatically presented as 24-hour graphs.

REMISSION OF DIABETES

Some patients with type 2 diabetes make significant lifestyle changes that result in the normalisation of their blood sugars and, indeed, lay media is full of advice on how people can 'cure' or 'reverse' their diabetes. However, because of the nature of the disease, defining a cure of diabetes has not been easy.[14] With an acute disease such as pneumonia or a fracture, the patient is either ill or cured, 'cure' meaning that the pathogen or underlying pathology is no longer present. But with a chronic disease such as diabetes, the pathologies underlying the disease are on a continuum; insulin resistance and pancreatic dysfunction may be minimal or excessive, and the expression of high blood sugars is dependent on the balance between the two. Normalisation of blood sugars occurs when the balance between the contributing pathologies is altered, i.e. blood sugars are normalised but neither pathology has necessarily been eradicated. Indeed, the person is at risk of relapse.

Based on an understanding that cure is defined as 'restoration to good health' with no chance of relapse, and remission defined as an 'abatement or disappearance of the signs and symptoms of a disease' with a risk of relapse, an expert advisory group for the American Diabetes Association has recommended that a person who has normalised blood sugars following a diagnosis of diabetes be regarded as in remission – not cured.[14] Of note, for a person to be in remission they must not be receiving treatment for diabetes. This means a person who has undergone gastric bypass surgery and has normalised blood sugars is not considered to be in remission.

Different levels of remission have been proposed based on how complete and for how long a person's

Table 8.1 Defining remission in diabetes[14]

Remission type	Definition	Management goals of comorbid conditions	Screening for microvascular disease
Partial	Hyperglycaemia below diagnostic threshold for diabetes but above normoglycaemia At least 1 year duration No pharmacologic therapy or ongoing procedures (i.e. gastric banding/ bypass)	Same as for patients *with* diabetes	Same as for patients *with* diabetes
Complete	Normoglycaemic blood sugars: 3.5–7.8 mmol/L (60–140 mL/dL) At least 1 year duration No pharmacologic therapy or ongoing procedures (i.e. gastric banding)	Same as for patients *with* diabetes	Same as for patients *with* diabetes
Prolonged	Complete remission for 5 years	Same as for patients *without* diabetes	Same as for patients *without* diabetes Only stop retinal/ renal screening if no previous history of it

blood sugars have been normalised (Table 8.1). Furthermore, as the pathologies contributing to elevated cardiovascular risk are still present following the normalisation of blood sugars, recommendations for ongoing screening and cardiovascular risk management for each level of remission have been provided.

It is important to remember (and to share with your patients) that not all people with type 2 diabetes will be able to achieve remission with lifestyle changes. Unlike those whose diabetes is predominantly due to insulin resistance, those whose diabetes is primarily due to pancreatic dysfunction will never be able to achieve remission, despite putting maximal effort into lifestyle changes.

SUMMARY

- It is essential that each patient understands the association between their HbA_{1c} and their cardiovascular risk/ long-term health.
- It is important that each patient understands what improvement in HbA_{1c} can be expected with each management choice.

- Patients should not be held to identical HbA_{1c} targets; glycaemic goals and frequency of checking HbA_{1c} should be individualised based on their cardiovascular risk and on their management regime.
- Self-monitoring of blood sugars should only be done if the resultant blood glucose value is going to contribute to management decision-making.
- Diabetes management decisions require a review of both the HbA_{1c} and the blood sugars. The HbA_{1c} tells us *whether* the person's management regime needs to be changed; blood sugar checks tell us *what* needs to be changed.
- Reading and interpreting blood sugars is an important skill to master and an important skill to teach patients.
- Remission of diabetes has been defined as normalisation of blood sugars in a patient not receiving any treatment. Three levels of remission have been proposed: partial, complete and prolonged.

REFERENCES

1. Stratton IM, Adler AI, Neil HAW, et al. Association of glycaemia with macrovascular and microvascular complications of type 2 diabetes (UKPDS 35): prospective observational study. BMJ. 2000;321:405–412

2. American Diabetes Association. Classification and diagnosis of diabetes: standards of medical care in diabetes – 2019. Diabetes Care. 2019;42(suppl1):S61–S70

3. Sherifali D, Nerenberg K, Pullenayegum E, et al. The effect of oral antidiabetic agents on A1C levels: a systematic review and meta-analysis. Diabetes Care. 2010;33(8):1859–1864

4. American Diabetes Association. Standards of medical care in diabetes – 2017. Diabetes Care. 2017;40(suppl1):S1–S135

5. Garber AJ, Abrahamson MJ, Barzilay JI, et al. Consensus statement by the American Association of Clinical Endocrinologists and American College of Endocrinology on the comprehensive type 2 diabetes management algorithm – 2016 executive summary. Endocr Pract. 2016;22:84–113

6. Gong S, Shuhua M, Hong T, et al. Association of glycemic variability and the presence and severity of coronary artery disease in patients with type 2 diabetes. Cardiovasc Diabetol. 2011;10:10–19

7. Agiostratidou G, Anhalt H, Ball D, et al. Standardizing clinically meaningful outcome measures beyond HbA$_{1c}$ for type 1 diabetes: a consensus report of the American Association of Clinical Endocrinologists, the American Association of Diabetes Educators, the American Diabetes Association, the Endocrine Society, JDRF International, The Leona M and Harry B Helmsley Charitable Trust, the Pediatric Endocrine Society, and the T1D Exchange. Diabetes Care. 2017;40:1622–1630

8. The Action to Control Cardiovascular Risk in Diabetes (ACCORD) Study Group. Effects of intensive glucose lowering in type 2 diabetes. N Engl J Med. 2008;358:2545–2559

9. The ADVANCE Collaborative Group. Intensive blood glucose control and vascular outcomes in patients with type 2 diabetes. N Engl J Med. 2008;358:2560–2572

10. Inzucchi SE, Bergenstal RM, Buse JB, et al. Management of hyperglycemia in type 2 diabetes: a patient-centered approach. Position statement of the American Diabetes Association (ADA) and the European Association for the Study of Diabetes (EASD). Diabetes Care. 2012;35:1364–1379

11. Hemmingsen B, Lund SS, Gluud C, et al. Intensive glycaemic control for patients with type 2 diabetes: systematic review with meta-analysis and trial sequential analysis of randomised clinical trials. BMJ. 2011;343:d6898

12. Howard-Thompson A, Khan M, Jones M, George CM. Type 2 diabetes mellitus: outpatient insulin management. Am Fam Phys. 2018;97:29–37

13. American Diabetes Association. Classification and diagnosis of diabetes: standards of medical care in diabetes – 2019. Diabetes Care. 2019;42(suppl1):S71–S80

14. Buse JB, Caprio S, Cefalu WT, et al. How do we define cure of diabetes? Diabetes Care. 2009;32:2133–2135

9

Lifestyle management

Lifestyle modification is an integral part of diabetes management regardless of the type of diabetes a person has. However, unfortunately, it is often only those with pre-diabetes or type 2 who receive education around lifestyle modification.[1] Of course, the reason for this is that, unlike genetic or auto-immune types of diabetes, newly diagnosed type 2 is considered potentially preventable through lifestyle modification.[2-4]

Three landmark studies using dietary and exercise intervention in people at high risk for developing type 2 diabetes demonstrated a 3- to 6-year delay in the progression to type 2 diabetes.[5-7] Weight loss,[8] lower HbA_{1c},[9] improved quality of life,[10] along with reductions in all-cause mortality[10] and healthcare costs[11] are also reported.

While weight loss, exercise and 'healthy' eating are all considered important components of lifestyle management, it is unclear which of these components is the most important. Some claim weight loss to be the most important.[12-17] Yet the remarkable remission of diabetes in those who receive gastric bypass surgery prior to losing any significant amounts of weight suggest dietary changes might be more important.[18]

Sadly, education for lifestyle management within a busy clinical setting often translates into the provider simply telling the patient to 'exercise more', or 'eat healthy'. However, simply telling someone they must exercise or change their eating habits rarely works. Indeed, while we have good evidence from controlled research settings supporting the need for education around lifestyle changes, there has been little success in our ability to establish inexpensive community-based interventions that produce long-term changes in people's lifestyle choices.

A patient-centred approach shifts away from telling people what to do, to focusing on providing the information and knowledge that will assist them with their everyday choices. Ensuring a person understands *how* exercise and food affect blood sugars is considered key to achieving long-term behavioural change.

To increase the likelihood of a person's both realising and adhering to lifestyle changes, the patient-centred provider may also need to take the time to find each person's internal motivator. Within the patient-centred framework this is referred to as 'finding common ground'. How to develop the patient-centred skills necessary for finding common ground is outlined in Chapter 11, Providing Patient-Centred Care, and will often require a return to the original diagram (Figure 1.2) to review how exercise and eating fit into the physiology of glucose metabolism.

EXERCISE

The positive benefits of exercise are extensive: improved cardiovascular health and better bone health along with a reduced risk of developing diabetes, obesity, sleep apnoea and cancer. There are also the psychosocial benefits of improved mood, improved mobility and independence.[19,20] As noted earlier, despite these universal benefits, discussions on the importance of exercise for someone with diabetes are typically reserved for the patients with type 2. While exercise for someone with type 1 diabetes does not improve the underlying pathological defect causing their disease, it can contribute to long-term improvements in glycaemic control and, just as importantly, helps to reduce the risk of obesity and all of the associated metabolic derangements often acquired in the latter years.

Exercise directly affects blood sugars by improving insulin sensitivity, which in turn improves long-term glycaemic control.[4,21] Regular physical activity reduces the risk of developing type 2 diabetes by 20–30%.[4–7,12,23,24] This improvement is independent of any change in body weight.[6,22]

There is no evidence to support one type of exercise over another. Both aerobic and resistance training generate improvements in insulin sensitivity that can last up to 72 hours.[20,25,26] Resistance training, which increases both muscle mass and endurance, has been shown to alter both body composition and improve glycaemic control more rapidly than aerobic training alone.[20] Accordingly, the current recommendations for people with diabetes are to participate in moderate-intensity aerobic exercise at 50–70% of maximum heart rate for 150 minutes per week with resistance exercises 3 days a week.[27]

Potential risks

Exercise in diabetes can be associated with risks, and healthcare providers should be familiar with who might be susceptible to adverse effects.[20] Comorbidities, diabetes complications, medications and physical limitations all need to be considered when a person is starting an exercise programme.

- **Retinopathy.** High-impact aerobic or heavy resistance exercises are not recommended in those with severe proliferative or non-proliferative retinopathy because of the risk of haemorrhage or retinal detachment.[28]
- **Peripheral neuropathy.** Reduced sensation in the lower extremity increases the risk of undetected skin breakdown and/or Charcot joint destruction. Thus, for those with severe peripheral neuropathy, non-weight-bearing activities such as swimming or cycling should be recommended. Weight-bearing exercise is contraindicated in someone with an active foot ulceration.[29]
- **Autonomic neuropathy.** A cardiac screen is recommended before beginning any exercise programme for people with autonomic neuropathy as they are likely to have underlying cardiovascular disease. Supervision during exercise is also suggested due to the risk of

hypotension, arrhythmias and hypoglycaemia secondary to gastroparesis and hypoglycaemic unawareness.[30]

- **Microalbuminuria.** Some recommend that people with renal disease limit themselves to light or moderate exercise as physical activity can cause an acute increase in urinary protein levels. However, there is no evidence that increased proteinuria from high-level exercise increases the rate of renal deterioration.[30]
- **Medication management.** As exercise directly affects blood sugars, it is essential that anyone with diabetes understands how exercising will influence their blood sugars and/or insulin doses. For those who have well-controlled diabetes and are on insulin or insulin secretagogues, blood sugar should be checked before and after exercise and, if the workout is extended, during exercise. Patients who are susceptible to hypoglycaemia or have hypoglycaemic unawareness should consider reducing their doses of medication or eat carbohydrate before they exercise.[31]

FOODS

As with exercise, ingestion of food directly affects blood sugars. Unlike exercise, however, eating is a completely indispensable activity of daily living; without it we would die. Except for a handful of foods (e.g. sugar-sweetened beverages), all foods contain nutrients that are advantageous. Furthermore, food plays an important role socially and culturally. A full review of nutritional recommendations for people with diabetes and pre-diabetes is beyond the scope of this manual but can be found elsewhere.[32] However, as foods clearly affect blood sugars and this is a manual about managing blood sugars, anyone with diabetes should be provided with accurate information on how different foods affect blood sugars differently and how to combine different foods to assist with blood sugar control.

Unfortunately, within the clinical setting, dietary 'education' is often reduced to telling people which are 'good' foods and which are 'bad'; or even worse, they are simply told to 'eat a healthy diet'. This not only presumes that the person knows what a healthy diet is, but also makes the erroneous assumption that foods can be divided into black and white categories of 'healthy' or 'not healthy', 'good' or 'bad'. As noted above, almost all foods have nutrients that are important for maintaining health. How 'healthy' a food actually is depends on what aspect of health is being considered; adhering to a high-fibre diet rich in fruit and whole grains is a 'healthy' or 'good' diet when considering the prevention of colon cancer. However, for someone with diabetes, such a diet would contribute to elevated blood sugars.

A patient-centred approach to dietary education provides no instruction on what the person should and should not eat. It simply provides information on how different foods affect blood sugars differently, and how different foods can be combined to minimise post-meal blood sugar spikes. Armed with this information, each person can then make their own well-informed decisions with regard to their diet. This approach allows for cultural and personal preferences and removes the guilt that is so often associated with eating so-called 'bad' foods. As I often point out to a patient, they actually can eat cake and have a normal blood sugar. This statement invariably piques their interest – as it has likely piqued yours – and I now have their attention for what is usually the most dreaded subject for many of those who have diabetes.

The following is the conversation that I have with patients when discussing foods. Obviously, the approach should be adapted to suit whoever is sitting in front of you. But, regardless of the approach taken, it is important that you provide the same information to every patient. Bear in mind that language used around food can often be emotive and judgemental. My advice would be to avoid words such as diet, good, bad, better, worse, naughty, and so on.

Foods have been divided into three different groups – carbohydrates, proteins and fats. Is this a concept that you are familiar with?

The reason foods have been divided into these three different groups is because there are three different ways that our body processes the food, breaking it down into nutrients we can use; carbohydrates follow one digestive process, proteins follow a completely different digestive process, while fats follow a third.

So, let's take a look at which foods belong in each category.

What kind of foods do you think of as carbohydrates? ..... proteins? .... fats?

Having the patient name the foods for each category ensures they are engaged and provides opportunity for them to mention the foods that they most often use. It also allows you to gauge the person's level of knowledge. While many have a reasonable understanding of food types, others do not and you will need to assist. Together, you will create a personalised chart that will look something like Patient Handout 9.

Now there are a number of foods we have not mentioned such as salad and vegetables. We will consider these later.

So, looking at the three food groups – which do you believe will raise your blood sugars when you eat them? Is it foods in all of the three groups, or is it only two of the groups – or only one?

Again, asking questions keeps the person engaged and interested.

Only one of these food groups raises our blood sugars when we eat them – the carbohydrates.[1] Proteins and fats do not immediately contribute to the rise in blood sugars. However, they do modify how high your blood sugars will go after a meal. Let's play a bit of a game to show you what I mean.

Let's say you woke up this morning and decided to have two slices of toast for breakfast – two slices of toast with nothing on them; essentially a pure carbohydrate meal. What happens to the blood sugars? First, because you are eating carbohydrate the blood sugars will rise and, because it is only carbohydrate being eaten, the blood sugars rise quite quickly, peak at about 30 minutes and then drop relatively quickly. In someone who does not have diabetes, the blood sugars will be back to baseline about 1.5 to 2 hours after eating (solid line, Figure 9.1).

The next morning you decide to have the same two slices of toast. However, this time you add some eggs. So, the meal is now a mixture of carbohydrate and protein. Again, because you are eating carbohydrate, the blood sugars will rise. Indeed, you are eating exactly the same amount of carbohydrate as you ate the previous morning (two slices of toast). However, because the protein is now added to the carbohydrate, the blood sugars do not rise quite so quickly and the peak is delayed. The peak also does not go so high, with the drop back to baseline taking longer – about 2–4 hours (dashed line, Figure 9.1).

So even though you ate the same two slices of toast, your blood sugar after the meal does not spike

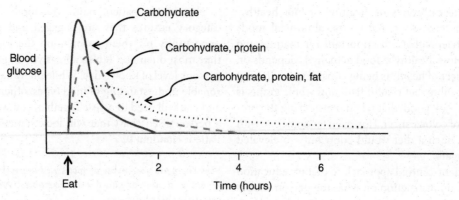

Figure 9.1 The effect of foods on post-meal blood glucose.

as high as it did when you ate the toast without the protein.

On the third morning, you again eat the same two slices of toast with the eggs but this time you add slathers of butter to the toast. The meal now contains food from all three food groups – carbohydrate, protein and fat. Once again, because you are eating carbohydrate, the blood sugars rise. However, with the fat added to the carbohydrate and protein, there is a further delay in the blood glucose spike after the meal, a further reduction in how high the blood sugars rise and the blood glucose drop back to baseline takes even longer – about 4–6 hours (dotted line, Figure 9.1).

So how do we translate this understanding into eating in a way that will help you to manage your blood sugars?

The first message is – shift away from thinking about foods as being good or bad. Indeed, we certainly don't want you to conclude that, as carbohydrates are responsible for raising blood sugars, they should be removed from your diet. Carbohydrates are valuable, nutritious foods and should be a part of anyone's diet. Furthermore, carbohydrates are the staple of any celebratory feast. So, to simply remove them from your meals is impractical, unrealistic and not a sensible solution. Having said that, there are two foods in the carbohydrate list that should be avoided – fizzy drinks (soda) and juice.

The second message is – foods such as leafy green vegetables and salad vegetables are carbohydrates but their carbohydrate content is minimal and they will contribute little to post-meal blood sugars. However, it is important to understand that they do not help to blunt the post-meal blood sugar spike. So, having a tomato and lettuce sandwich will produce the same post-meal blood sugar has eating

the bread on its own. To better manage blood sugars, cheese or some other protein should be added to the tomato and lettuce.

The third message is – as carbohydrates are going to be a part of most if not all your meals, be sure to always eat them along with proteins and fats to minimise the post-meal sugar spike. The idea is not to remove carbohydrates, but reduce the carbohydrate proportion of the meal, relative to the protein and fats proportions. If making a cake for a special occasion, make a cream cheese icing and sprinkle nuts on top. Approach each meal with the idea of 'mixing and matching' your foods – if dessert is being offered, hold back on the potato in the main course.

Other examples of 'mixing and matching' to minimise blood sugars spikes are:

- Choose a peanut butter sandwich, not a banana sandwich or a jam sandwich.
- Add cheese to your tomato sandwich.
- Don't put sweet potato, mashed potato, yams, corn and peas all in the same meal. Combine the sweet potato with broccoli and carrots in one meal, save the yams for another.
- If ice cream is on the menu, serve it up in a dish not in a cone. Put some nuts on top.
- Nibble on nuts rather than crisps (chips). If you are going to have crisps, dunk them in the dip. If you are going to have crackers, eat them with cheese.
- Avoid the foods in the supermarket that are labelled as low fat. When the fat is removed food does not taste so good. To improve on the taste, manufacturers often add thickeners and sugars (both carbohydrates). Thus, ice cream (made with real cream) would be a better choice than low-fat frozen yoghurt or water ice.

- *There is nothing wrong with eating a takeaway meal if the right menu choices are made. A McDonald's hamburger contains macronutrients from all three food groups. What is wrong with takeaways? It is the slushies, the fries and the fizzy drinks that accompany the meal. Fish and chips night for the family does not need to be given up, simply opt to replace the chips with a serving of onion rings.*

If your patient has a blood glucose meter, encourage them to experiment. Suggest they check their blood sugar prior to eating a favourite meal that is carbohydrate heavy and then repeat the blood sugar check 30–60 minutes later. Provide recommendations as to how the relative proportions of carbohydrate/protein/fat in the meal can be altered and have them repeat the exercise.

Many studies have attempted to identify the optimal proportions of carbohydrates, proteins and fats for people with diabetes, but no optimal combination has been found. However, "reducing overall carbohydrate intake for individuals with diabetes has demonstrated the most evidence for improving glycemia and may be applied in a variety of eating patterns that meet individual needs and preferences."[32] Thus, our approach to portion control is to suggest that the person simply focus on reducing their carbohydrate intake less than 50 g per meal.

Other important educational points to cover:

- Ensure the person understands that all carbohydrates are sugars.
- Explain that the delay and blunting of the post-meal blood sugar spike following mixed meals is the result of a slowed digestive process that delays glucose absorption. Digestion of carbohydrates begins immediately in the mouth and, if they are eaten on their own, they can be absorbed directly into the bloodstream under the tongue. When eaten with protein and fat, the carbohydrate is not digested until it reaches the stomach, where the protein and fat are mixed with it. This delay in the digestive process slows the absorption of the carbohydrate into the bloodstream. This is why simple sugars such as juice, fizzy drinks and the modern day smoothie (which eliminates the digestive process) produce immediate blood sugar spikes.

- Be sure the person understands how to read a food label, emphasising the need to look at 'total carbohydrates' as opposed to 'sugars' when considering how the food will influence their blood sugars.
- Ensure the person understands that fat and cholesterol are essential for normal bodily functions. Keep in mind that studies have provided inconclusive findings with regard to the role dietary cholesterol plays, if any, in blood cholesterol levels and cardiovascular events in people with diabetes.[32,34,35]
- There is no evidence that eating foods with low glycaemic index will change clinically relevant outcomes such as HbA_{1c}, morbidity or mortality.[36] Further, studies have found little difference in glycaemic excursions when comparing ingestion of foods with a high glycaemic index versus a low glycaemic index. Thus, eating white rice will produce a similar glucose excursion to eating brown rice.
- There has been a great deal of interest in using micronutrients such as chromium and zinc, antioxidants and herbal supplements to improve diabetes control. Although some small studies have suggested a benefit from chromium, other studies and meta-analyses have not reached the same conclusion. Currently there are no large, well-controlled studies that prove the benefit of specific micronutrients in the management of diabetes.[37]

SUMMARY

- Lifestyle modification is an integral part of diabetes management, regardless of the type of diabetes a person has.
- The positive benefits of exercise are extensive, both medically and psychosocially.
- Both aerobic and resistance exercise reduce blood glucose by increasing insulin sensitivity. Exercise also contributes to weight loss, which further increases insulin sensitivity. To be of benefit, a person should exercise every 2–3 days.

- Exercise in those with diabetes can be associated with risks, and healthcare providers should be familiar with the comorbidities, diabetes complications and medications that can impact exercise participation.
- Foods are categorised into three different food groups (carbohydrates, protein and fats), each food group requiring a different digestive pathway.
- Anyone with diabetes should be provided with information on how different foods affect blood sugars differently and how to combine different foods to assist with blood sugar control.

NOTE

1 In people with type 1 diabetes protein consumption can contribute to an immediate elevation of blood sugars. However, in people with type 2 diabetes protein consumption does not.[33]

REFERENCES

1. Gonder-Frederick L. Lifestyle modifications in the management of type 1 diabetes: still relevant after all these years? Diabetes Technol Ther. 2014;16:695–698
2. Jakicic JM, Jaramilo SA, Balasubramanyam A, et al. Effect of a lifestyle intervention on change in cardiorespiratory fitness in adults with type 2 diabetes: results from the Look AHEAD study. Int J Obes (Lond). 2009;33:305–316
3. O'Gorman DJ, Krook A. Exercise and the treatment of diabetes and obesity. Endocrinol Metab Clin North Am. 2008;37:887–903
4. Gill JM, Cooper AR. Physical activity and prevention of type 2 diabetes mellitus. Sports Med. 2008;38:806–824
5. Pan XR, Li GW, Hu YH, et al. Effects of diet and exercise in preventing NIDDM in people with impaired glucose tolerance. The Da Qing IGT and Diabetes Study. Diabetes Care. 1997;20:537–544
6. Tuomilehto J, Lindstrom J, Eriksson JG, et al.; the Finnish Diabetes Prevention Study Group. Prevention of type 2 diabetes mellitus by changes in lifestyle among subjects with impaired glucose tolerance. N Engl J Med. 2001;344:1343–1350
7. Diabetes Prevention Program Research Group. Reduction in the incidence of type 2 diabetes with lifestyle intervention or metformin. N Engl J Med. 2002;346:393–403
8. Steinsbekk A, Rygg LO, Lisulo M, et al. Group based diabetes self-management education compared to routine treatment for people with type 2 diabetes mellitus. A systematic review with meta-analysis. BMC Health Serv Res. 2012;12:213
9. Norris SL, Lau J, Smith SJ, et al. Self-management education for adults with type 2 diabetes: a meta-analysis of the effect on glycemic control. Diabetes Care. 2002;25;1159–1171
10. Cochran J, Conn VS. Meta-analysis of quality of life outcomes following diabetes self-management training. Diabetes Educ. 2008;34:815–823
11. Duncan I, Ahmed T, Li QE, et al. Assessing the value of the diabetes educator. Diabetes Educ. 2011;37:638–657
12. Eakin EG, Reeves MM, Lawler SP, et al. The Logan Healthy Living Program: a cluster randomized trial of a telephone-delivered physical activity and dietary behavior intervention for primary care patients with type 2 diabetes for hypertension from a socially disadvantaged community: rationale, design and recruitment. Contemp Clin Trials. 2008;29:439–454
13. Amati F, Barthassat V, Miganne G, et al. Enhancing regular physical activity and relapse prevention through a 1-day therapeutic patient education workshop: a pilot study. Patient Educ Couns. 2007;68:70–78
14. Bo S, Ciccone G, Baldi C, et al. Effectiveness of a lifestyle intervention on metabolic syndrome: a randomized controlled trial. J Gen Intern Med. 2007:22:1695–1703
15. Dunstan DW, Vulikh E, Owen N, et al. Community center-based resistance training for the maintenance of glycemic control in adults with type 2 diabetes. Diabetes Care. 2006;29:2586–2591
16. Sigal RJ, Kenny GP, Boule NG, et al. Effects of aerobic training, resistance training or both on glycemic control in type 2 diabetes: a randomized trial. Ann Intern Med. 2007;147:357–369
17. Aylin K, Arzu D, Sabri S, et al. The effect of combined resistance and home-based walking exercise in type 2 diabetes patients. Int J Diabetes Dev Ctries. 2009;29:159–165

18. Dixon JB, O'Brien PE, Playfair J, et al. Adjustable gastric banding and conventional therapy for type 2 diabetes: a randomized controlled trial. JAMA. 2008;299:316–323

19. Nordmann AJ, Nordmann A, Briel M, et al. Effects of low-carbohydrate vs low-fat diets on weight loss and cardiovascular risk factors: a meta-analysis of randomized controlled trials. Arch Intern Med. 2006;166:285–293

20. Green DS, Mandarino LJ, Pendergrass M. Exercise in diabetes. In Fonseca VA (ed) Clinical diabetes: translating research into practice. Saunders Elsevier, Philadelphia, 2006

21. Qi L, Hu FB, Hu G. Genes, environment and interactions in prevention of type 2 diabetes: a focus on physical activity and lifestyle changes. Curr Mol Med. 2008;8:519–532

22. Boule N, Haddad E, Kenny GP, et al. Effects of exercise on glycemic control and body mass in type 2 diabetes mellitus: a meta-analysis of controlled clinical trials. JAMA. 2001;286:1218–1227

23. Hu FB, Sigal RJ, Rich-Edwards JW, et al. Walking compared with vigorous physical activity and risk of type 2 diabetes in women. JAMA. 1999;282:1433–1439

24. Helmrich SP, Ragland DR, Leung RW, Paffengerger RS. Physical activity and reduced occurrence of non-insulin-dependent diabetes mellitus. N Engl J Med. 1991;325:147–152

25. Ivy JL. Role of exercise training in the prevention and treatment of insulin resistance and non-insulin dependent diabetes mellitus. Sports Med. 1997;24:321–336

26. Wallberg-Henriksson H, Rincon J, Zierath JR. Exercise in the management of non-insulin-dependent diabetes mellitus. Sports Med. 1998;25:25–35

27. Sigal RJ, Kenny JP, Wasserman DH, Castaneda-Sceppa C. Physical activity/exercise and type 2 diabetes. Diabetes Care. 2004;27:2518–2539

28. Aiello LP, Wong J, Cavallerano JD, et al. Retinopathy. In Ruderman N, Devlin JT, Schneider SH, Kriska A (eds) Handbook on exercise in diabetes, 2nd ed. American Diabetes Association, Alexandria VA, 2002, pp 401–413

29. Levin ME. The diabetic foot. In Ruderman N, Devlin JT, Schneider SH, Kriska A (eds) Handbook on exercise in diabetes, 2nd ed. American Diabetes Association, Alexandria VA, 2002, pp 385–399

30. Colberg SR, Sigal RJ, Yardley JE, et al. Physical activity/exercise and diabetes: a position statement of the American Diabetes Association. Diabetes Care. 2016;39:2065–2079

31. Berger M. Adjustment of insulin and oral agent therapy. In Ruderman N, Devlin JT, Schneider SH, Kriska A (eds) Handbook on exercise in diabetes, 2nd ed. American Diabetes Association, Alexandria VA, 2002, pp 365–376

32. Evert AB, Dennison M, Gardner CD, et al. Nutrition therapy for adults with diabetes or prediabetes: a consensus report. Diabetes Care. 2019;42:731–754

33. Gannon MC, Nuttall JA, Damberg G, et al. Effect of protein ingestion on the glucose appearance rate in people with type 2 diabetes. J Clin Endocrinol Metab. 2001;86:1040–1047

34. Haffner SM, Lehto S, Tonnemaa T, et al. Mortality from coronary heart disease in subjects with type 2 diabetes and in nondiabetic subjects with and without prior myocardial infarction. N Engl J Med. 1998;339:229–234

35. Taubes G. Why we get fat and what to do about it. Anchor Books, Random House, NY, 2010

36. Vega-Lopez s, Venn BJ, Slavin JL. Relevance of the glycemic index and glyemic load for body weight, diabetes, and cardiovascular disease. Nutrients. 2018;10:1361

37. American Diabetes Association. Nutrition recommendations and interventions for diabetes [position statement]. Diabetes Care. 2007;30(suppl1):S48–S65

10

Cardiovascular risk management

Many people, including providers, see diabetes simply as a disease of high sugars and that, as such, the management of diabetes is about minimising hyperglycaemia. In truth, however, it would be more appropriate to think of diabetes as a vascular disease placing a person with diabetes at high risk for cardiovascular events.

From this broader perspective, management shifts from the narrow focus of blood glucose control to the broader, more clinically relevant focus of minimising cardiovascular risk. Indeed, focusing on glycaemic control alone has little impact on reducing a person's overall cardiovascular risk, and the long-practiced glucocentric approach to diabetes management is no longer considered acceptable.[1] To obtain clinically meaningful improvements in cardiovascular risk, diabetes care must include comprehensive management of five clinical parameters: glycaemia, blood pressure, cholesterol, body weight and smoking. Each parameter contributes independently to a person's cardiovascular risk and, as such, each has a recommended 'gold standard' target for minimising its contribution to cardiovascular risk (Table 10.1) – albeit with emphasis on the need to individualise these targets according to the medico-psychosocial complexity of each patient.[2]

Other factors also contribute to a person's cardiovascular risk, including ethnicity, family history of cardiovascular disease and number of years with diabetes. To assist with risk stratification of patients, algorithms that incorporate clinical and ethnic parameters have been developed. One of the first algorithms for calculating cardiovascular risk was the Framingham Risk Score.[3] However, many others have since been developed, including ones tailored for use within specific countries.

Being able to define a person's cardiovascular risk has improved our ability to assess the benefits and risks of intensifying medical management. Introducing medications to tighten clinical parameters is not without risk and, indeed, may not provide additional benefit. This was clearly demonstrated in the ADVANCE[4] and ACCORD[5] trials. Each study took a large population of people with diabetes and attempted to drive their HbA_{1c} to < 48 mmol/mol (6.5%). Unexpectedly, for some participants, these attempts to tighten the HbA_{1c} resulted in increased cardiovascular events and all-cause mortality, forcing us to reassess recommendations around HbA_{1c} targets.

Managing cardiovascular risk invariably requires people with diabetes to take multiple medications every day. As we are all aware, achieving this endpoint can be a considerable challenge. Indeed, one study found each increase in the number of blood pressure pills prescribed resulted in an 80% increase in risk for non-adherence.[6] To support successful daily decision-making around self-management, each person must be well informed, not just about cardiovascular risk in general, but about *their* cardiovascular risk. Patients presented with personalised risk information are more likely to make informed decisions than patients who are presented with generic risk information.[7] For example, do not just tell a patient they will go blind if they do not manage their diabetes – review what retinopathy actually is (vascular damage), review their actual retinal screen results and discuss their risk of further disease based on their current HbA_{1c}. Patient Handouts have been provided at the end of this manual to help support these educational discussions.

Table 10.1 Gold standard targets for managing cardiovascular risk[2]

Diabetes	$HbA_{1c} \leq 48$ mmol/mol (6.5%)
Hypertension	Blood pressure < 140/90
Cholesterol	LDL < 1.8 mmol/L (70 mg/dL)
Smoking	None
Weight	Body mass index (weight in kg/height in m^2) ≤ 25

Supporting fully informed decision-making will also require an explanation as to how each risk factor contributes physiologically to cardiovascular risk and how management choice can minimise this contribution. These explanations need to be comprehensive and tailored to the educational level of each individual. Unfortunately, attempts to simplify medical information often result in the omission of details. Once this happens, the patient is no longer fully informed, and daily self-management decisions are less likely to result in appropriate choices.

Thus, it is important that every provider have a set of 'tools', each tool being a comprehensive, detailed but simple explanation for the pathology and management of each cardiovascular risk parameter. Below (in *italic*) I describe some of the 'tools' I have created and found to work well. Each can be covered in a 3- to 5-minute conversation during a busy clinic and, more often than not, each produces the desired long-term behavioural change in patient self-management we are striving for. Patient Handout 10 can be used to support these conversations.

DIABETES

When helping a person to manage their diabetes a great deal of time is spent focusing on blood glucose control and the need to get the HbA_{1c} to target. It is easy, in all this effort, to forget about bringing the patient into the bigger picture so they understand exactly what the HbA_{1c} is measuring and what information it is giving us around their cardiovascular risk. Providing this information more often than not achieves the patient-centred requisite 'finding common ground' (see Chapter 11, Providing Patient-Centred Care) as, following the explanation, the patient often asks, "What can I do to get my HbA_{1c} down?" Indeed, the following

has consistently been my most successful tool for achieving long-term changes in patient behaviour.

Every 3 months or so, you are sent for some blood tests – do you know what these blood tests are checking?

One of the blood tests is your HbA_{1c}. Is this a term you are familiar with?

The HbA_{1c} gives us two very valuable pieces of information. What is your understanding of what the HbA_{1c} tells us?

Remember that asking questions both engages the person and provides you with information about the person's current level of understanding.

Before we talk about what information the HbA_{1c} provides, let me explain what this blood test is actually measuring. We have talked about how glucose is our fuel and how it is transported to all parts of our body within the blood vessels. Glucose, of course, is not the only thing that is in our blood; we have red blood cells, white blood cells, water and cholesterol amongst other things. As the glucose travels in the blood vessels, it 'sticks' to everything. Thus, as the red blood cells, which have nothing to do with diabetes, roll along in the blood vessels, the glucose sticks to the outside of them – a bit like rolling biscuit dough in coconut (Figure 10.1). The sugar sticking to the outside of the red blood cells happens in everyone whether they have diabetes or not, because we all have red blood cells and we all have glucose in our blood. However, as you can imagine, if the blood has a higher content of glucose (i.e. the person has diabetes), then more of the outside surface of the red blood cells will be covered in sugar.

We have a way of measuring how much of the surface of your red blood cells is covered with glucose – and that is your HbA_{1c}.

In a person who does not have diabetes, about 5% of the surface of the red blood cells is covered with sugar. In other words, their HbA_{1c} is 5%.

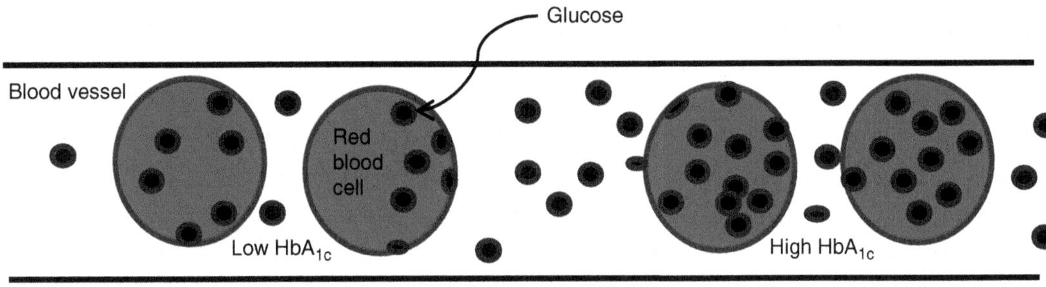

Figure 10.1 HbA_{1c} measures how much of the surface of the red blood cell is covered with glucose (glycated).

Your red blood cells are covered by ....% – or in other words your HbA_{1c} is ....

This HbA_{1c} gives us two pieces of information. First, it provides information about what your blood sugars have been. We have a chart (Patient Handouts 2 and 3) that translates the HbA_{1c} into what your average blood sugar has been for the past 3 months.

The HbA_{1c} reflects 3 months of your blood sugars because the lifespan of a red blood cell is 3 months. After 3 months, each red blood cell is removed from circulation and replaced with a new, clean one with no sugar stuck on the outside. This new red blood cell then rolls around for 3 months gathering sugars. So, every 3 months we have a complete turnover of our red blood cells. This is why you are asked to do blood tests every 3 months.

But there is a second piece of information that the HbA_{1c} gives us – perhaps a more important piece of information. Your HbA_{1c} tells us how likely you are to have a heart attack or stroke within the next year. We know from studies that for every 1% point you lower your HbA_{1c}, your risk of having a heart attack or stroke is reduced by 27% per year.[8-10]

Now your HbA_{1c} is ....

So, your risk of having a heart attack or stroke within the next year is ....

IN COUNTRIES WHERE HBA_{1c} IS NO LONGER REPORTED AS A PERCENTAGE

We no longer report HbA_{1c} as a percentage. We have gone metric. Just as we went from inches to centimetres we have gone from percentages to mmol/mol. We are still measuring how much sugar is stuck on the outside of the red blood cells, but we are reporting different numbers. As you can see from the chart (Patient Handout 2), your HbA_{1c} is ...... mmol/mol.

The important thing to remember is that a 1% point drop in your HbA_{1c} is equivalent to a drop of 11 mmol/mol. So, for every 10 mmol/mol that you reduce your HbA_{1c}, your risk of a heart attack or stroke will be reduced by 27% per year.

Now, I imagine that at some time you have been told that if you do not take care of your diabetes you will not only have a heart attack or stroke but may also "go blind", "lose your toes" or "end up on renal dialysis". So, what is it about diabetes that causes problems to happen all over our body?

Remember how we mentioned earlier that the sugar in the blood sticks everywhere. Well, one of the places that it sticks is on the inside of the blood vessel walls. This damages the walls. Once again, this happens in all of us whether we have diabetes or not, as we all have sugar in our blood. Fortunately, our bodies repair the damage. However, you can imagine that if a person has high sugars, then more will stick on the inside of the blood vessel walls and more damage will occur. The repair process is unable to keep up and over time the blood vessels are destroyed. Now, the large blood vessels don't do too badly and blood can continue to flow. However, the tiny blood vessels don't do so well and over time they are destroyed. So, diabetes is a disease of the tiny blood vessels.

Where are the tiny blood vessels in our body? They are in the brain, the eyes, the heart, the kidneys, and some of the tiniest blood vessels are wrapped around the pain nerves in our toes. So this is why poorly controlled diabetes causes dementia, strokes, blindness, heart attacks, pain in the legs and amputations. Indeed, for every 10 mmol/mol (1% point) that you reduce your HbA_{1c}, you reduce the risk of destroying your tiny blood vessels by 22% per year.[8-10]

BLOOD PRESSURE

When your blood pressure is checked, two numbers are recorded. Each number gives us specific information about how your heart is working.

The heart is a big muscle that sits in your chest. It is hollow and contains blood. When the heart muscle contracts, it squeezes the blood out of the heart into the blood vessels and around the body. We can measure the pressure in the blood vessels in much the same way we measure the pressure in car tyres. When a healthy heart contracts, the pressure in the blood vessels is around 120 mmHg. This is the top number in a recorded blood pressure.

After a contraction the heart muscle relaxes. This allows the heart to fill up with blood ready for the next contraction. During this relaxation phase, we can also measure the pressure in the blood vessels. In a healthy heart the pressure during this relaxation phase is around 80 mmHg. This is the bottom number in a recorded blood pressure.

So, the top number tells us how hard the heart is working when it is contracting while the bottom number tells us how well the heart is relaxing. Normal blood pressure in a healthy adult is generally around 120/80 mmHg, and any blood pressure less than 140/90 mmHg is considered normal.

Your two numbers are ....

If, for some reason, the heart has to work hard to squeeze the blood out, then the pressure in the blood vessels will increase and the top number of the recorded blood pressure will be elevated. If the heart is forced to do this over a period of time the heart muscle will get bigger, just like any other hardworking muscle in the body would. As the heart gets bigger, its muscle walls get thicker, and as they get thicker they get stiffer. As a stiff muscle will not relax very well, the pressure in the blood vessels during relaxation will rise and the bottom number of the recorded blood pressure will rise. Furthermore, if the heart is not relaxing well, it will not be filling very well, so now the heart will have to beat faster to ensure that the body continues get the blood it requires. So, the heart is now working even harder. It is not difficult to see that a vicious cycle is set up – a faster heart will be working harder, will get larger, stiffer, will have to beat faster and work even harder. This eventually leads to heart failure.

Another problem with the heart muscle wall becoming thicker is that the tiny blood vessels that feed the heart muscle are no longer able to cope with the increased needs of the larger muscle mass. When the heart muscle wall is not provided with sufficient blood, a heart attack will occur.

So, the two numbers in your blood pressure tell us a lot about how much your heart is working. Let's take another look at your numbers ....

One final point: up until now we have spent a great deal of time talking about managing your blood sugars. However, when it comes to managing your cardiovascular risk, it is far more important to have your blood pressure well controlled than it is to have your blood sugars well controlled.

CHOLESTEROL

Understanding cholesterol can be quite confusing as there are many different kinds. There is total cholesterol, LDL, HDL, triglycerides and more. Cholesterol is an essential nutrient for the body, with most of it (about two-thirds) made in the liver; the rest is obtained from diet.

Most of us think of cholesterol as being a problem because it builds up on the inside of our blood vessel walls. This cholesterol plaque, as we call it, narrows the blood vessels, making it harder for the heart to pump the blood around the body, i.e. cholesterol build-up increases blood pressure. If the cholesterol plaque builds up a lot, it can become quite unstable and bits of plaque can flick off, travel downstream in the blood and lodge in smaller blood vessels, blocking off the blood supply. If this occurs in the heart or brain, the person experiences a heart attack or stroke. Cholesterol build-up also disrupts the regular flow of blood. When blood flows irregularly, blood clots can form. These, like the bits of plaque, can sail off downstream and lodge in smaller blood vessels, again increasing the risk of having a heart attack or stroke.

It is the LDL cholesterol that is mostly responsible for cholesterol build-up. So, no surprise that the LDL is often referred to as the 'bad cholesterol'. For someone with diabetes, the current recommendation for minimising cardiovascular risk is to keep LDL less than 1.8 mmol/L (70 mg/dL).

Your LDL is ....

In contrast, the HDL cholesterol removes cholesterol from the blood vessel walls. For obvious reasons, it is referred to as the 'good cholesterol' and the goal is to have it as high as possible. An HDL greater than 1 mmol/L (40 mg/dL) is desirable.

Your HDL is ....

Clearly, as diabetes is a disease that damages blood vessels and puts you at high risk for heart attacks and strokes, it would be ideal to have your LDL as low as possible and your HDL as high as possible. To assist with this, the current recommendation is for people with diabetes to take *a medication called a statin. Statins have been shown to significantly reduce cardiovascular risk as they not only reduce the LDL but also stabilise the cholesterol plaques, prevent blood clots from forming and reduce inflammation and blood vessel damage.*

Thus, the recommendation for you would be to take ....

It is also important, of course, to review the possible side effects of statins.

Statins are the medication of choice for management of cholesterol.[2] Moderate-dose statins are recommended for anyone over the age of 40 with diabetes. Moderate-dose statins are also recommended for people under the age of 40 with diabetes and a cardiovascular risk of 20% over the next 20 years. High-dose statins are recommended for those over 40 with diabetes and a cardiovascular risk greater than 20% over the next 20 years.[2]

SMOKING

As always, the goal of a patient-centred encounter is to provide specific information about how smoking contributes to cardiovascular risk by raising blood pressure and causing vascular damage. However, I find a conversation around the cost of cigarettes is often more persuasive – especially if a person is weighing up the costs of a gym membership or they have a desirable item on their shopping wish list. Reviewing a handout like the one below is invaluable.

HOW MUCH OF YOUR MONEY HAS GONE UP IN SMOKE?[1]						
No. of cigarettes @ $40/pack	1 week	1 month	1 year	5 years	10 years	30 years
5 cigs/day (¼ pack)	$70	$300	$3,650	$18,250	$36,500	$109,500
10 cigs/day (½ pack)	$140	$600	$7,300	$36,500	$73,000	$219,000
20 cigs/day (1 pack)	$280	$1,200	$14,600	$73,000	$146,000	$438,000

WEIGHT

Obesity directly contributes to cardiovascular risk; it is associated with insulin resistance, high LDL, low HDL, increased inflammatory markers, sleep apnoea and reduced exercise. Thus, weight loss is recommended for all overweight or obese individuals who have or are at risk for diabetes.[2] However, there is no consensus on what the best way to lose weight is.

Furthermore, given obesity's multifactorial contributions to cardiovascular risk, it would be a complex task to tease out and then explain the many reasons why losing weight would be beneficial to someone with diabetes. One way of communicating obesity's contribution to cardiovascular risk is to simply point out that the heart in a person with a bigger body is likely to be working harder than the heart in a person with a smaller body. While oversimplistic and perhaps not entirely accurate, it certainly provides an easily grasped concept.

Fortunately, for the majority of the population being overweight is generally considered undesirable. Indeed, many are much more interested in losing weight than lowering blood sugars. So, unlike other cardiovascular risk factors, convincing a person on the need to lose weight is often not necessary. Of course, how to get the person to lose weight is the challenge – a challenge well suited to the provider skills reviewed in Chapter 11, Providing Patient-Centred Care.

RENAL PROTECTION

Think of your kidneys as sieves, filtering waste from the blood. Every time the heart pumps blood around your body, it goes through the kidneys, and any waste, excess water or other unneeded nutrients pass from the blood vessel through the 'sieve' and eventually end up in the urine. High sugars and high blood pressure damage the sieve; when it is damaged, it leaks, so that small proteins from your blood end up in the urine. We call this 'microalbuminuria', which is really just a fancy word meaning 'small protein in the urine'.

Microalbuminuria can be one of the first signs of kidney damage.

Sometimes when you are having your bloods done, you are asked to pee into a cup. This is to check if there are any proteins leaking into your urine.

The result from your most recent urine check is ....

If blood sugars and/or blood pressure remain high, the kidneys become increasingly damaged, the amount of protein in your urine increases and overall kidney function will begin to decline. Eventually, the kidneys' function may decline so much they can no longer filter out the unwanted contents of the blood, and renal dialysis (where a machine does the work of the kidneys) becomes necessary.

Obviously, keeping both your blood glucose and your blood pressure under good control will prevent or minimise damage to your kidneys. Indeed, if someone does have microalbuminuria, keeping blood sugars and blood pressure under control is essential if ongoing kidney function is to be preserved. Kidneys can be further protected from damage if a medication called an ACE or an ARB is taken. While we don't completely understand how these medications protect the kidneys, we do know that for maximal kidney protection the medication should be pushed up to maximum dose.

I will often point out to the patient, especially if they do not have any microalbuminuria, that ACEs (angiotensin-converting enzyme inhibitors) and ARBs (angiotensin receptor blockers) are also used for blood pressure control; indeed, they are considered the first-choice medication for blood pressure control in people with diabetes. However, to date, there is no evidence to support the addition of an ACE or an ARB for renal protection in a person with no hypertension and no microalbuminuria.

ASPIRIN USE

Aspirin inhibits blood clot formation, reducing the risk of heart attacks and strokes. Taking an aspirin a day is recommended for those with diabetes who have an increased cardiovascular risk (10-year risk > 10%).

Currently your overall cardiovascular risk is .... This is why aspirin has/has not been prescribed for you.

Of note, a 10-year cardiovascular risk greater than 10% includes most men who are older than 50 and most women who are older than 60 who have diabetes *and* one other major risk factor such as family history of a heart attack or stroke, high blood pressure, history of smoking, high LDL or microalbuminuria. Aspirin is not currently recommended for cardiovascular prevention in adults with diabetes who are at a low cardiovascular risk (10-year risk < 5%) as the risk of a stomach bleed outweighs any potential benefits.[2]

SUMMARY

- Managing diabetes is more than just managing blood sugars; it is about minimising cardiovascular risk. This requires monitoring and managing cholesterol, blood pressure, weight and smoking as well as introducing renal protection, if needed.
- Aiming for universal 'gold standard' targets for everyone with diabetes is no longer considered best practice. Targets should be individualised, taking into account overall cardiovascular risk, age of the patient, medication use and psychosocial situation.
- Patients presented with personalised risk information are more likely to make informed decisions about their personal cardiovascular risk management than patients who are presented with generic risk information.
- It is important that every provider have comprehensive, detailed but simple explanations for the pathology and management of each cardiovascular risk parameter.

NOTE

1 Figures based on the cost of one packet of cigarettes in New Zealand dollars in 2019, but the principle is the same in all countries. In 2019, NZ$40 equated to approximately UK£20 or US$26.

REFERENCES

1. Schernthaner G, Barnett AH, Betteridge DJ, et al. Is the ADA/EASD algorithm for the management of type 2 diabetes (January 2009) based on evidence or opinion? A critical analysis. Diabetologia. 2010;53:1258–1269

2. American Diabetes Association. Cardiovascular disease and risk management: standards of medical care in diabetes – 2019. Diabetes Care. 2019;42(suppl1):S103–S123

3. D'Agostino RB Sr, Vasan RS, Pencina MJ, et al. General cardiovascular risk profile for use in primary care: the Framingham Heart Study. Circulation. 2008;117: 743–753

4. The ADVANCE Collaborative Group. Intensive blood glucose control and vascular outcomes in patients with type 2 diabetes. N Engl J Med. 2008;358:2560–2572

5. The Action to Control Cardiovascular Risk in Diabetes Study Group. Effects of intensive glucose lowering in type 2 diabetes. N Engl J Med. 2008;358:2545–2559

6. Gupta P, Patel P, Horne R, et al. How to screen for non-adherence to antihypertensive therapy. Curr Hypertens. 2017;69:1113–1120

7. Edwards AG, Naik G, Ahmed H, et al. Personalised risk communication for informed decision making about taking screening tests. Cochrane Database Syst Rev. 2013;(2):CD001865

8. Diabetes Control and Complications Trial Research Group. The effect of intensive treatment of diabetes on the development and progression of long-term complications in insulin-dependent diabetes mellitus. N Engl J Med. 1993;329:977–986

9. UK Prospective Diabetes Study Group. Intensive blood-glucose control with sulphonylureas or insulin compared with conventional treatment and risk of complications in patients with type 2 diabetes. Lancet. 1998;352:837–853

10. Stratton IM, Adler AI, Neil HAW, et al. Association of glycaemia with macrovascular and microvascular complications of type 2 diabetes (UKPDS 35): prospective observational study. BMJ. 2000;321:405–412

11

Providing patient-centred care

"'True north' for quality care"

Club Diabete Sicili. Five-year impact of a continuous quality improvement effort implemented by a network of diabetes outpatient clinics. Diabetes Care. 2008;31:57–62

The current conventional model of healthcare has evolved to manage acute episodic illness and is ill-suited to approaching the complexities of chronic disease. With an acute disease event (e.g. a heart attack), healthcare providers must act quickly and decisively to save lives. During such events, while patients may be informed about what is happening, little time is dedicated to patient education regarding the disease process (e.g. plaque rupture) or treatment options – especially if the event is immediately life-threatening. The clinician is clearly in charge, and the patient surrenders autonomy to allow life-saving treatment to proceed rapidly. This provider-centred clinical decision-making has been further reinforced by the introduction of evidence-based clinical guidelines. Hospital clinicians are expected to follow very tight protocols for any number of acute life-threatening events, and wandering from a protocol could be considered the equivalent of committing medico-legal suicide.

With the advent of chronic disease, this kind of standardised approach to hospital (acute) disease management has been broadened to include preventative and chronic disease care. Expert panels representing various professional groups are continually updating the medical literature with evidence-based guidelines to assist with the prevention or management of long-term conditions. Guided by these protocols, the clinician's role is to monitor the disease and decide when treatment must be altered; the patient is a passive recipient of care who only needs to comply with what he/she is told,[1] and education, if considered necessary, is about 'helping' the patient to comply with the treatment guidelines.

There is no better example of this than the current approach to diabetes care. As providers, we are trained to determine what type of diabetes a person has; the type of diabetes then dictates the management approach. If the patient has type 1 diabetes, insulin is initiated. Initial management is with a fixed regime with set doses of insulin; a flexible regime, where the patient adjusts their insulin doses according to exercise and food consumption, is generally not introduced until later, if at all. Whether it is introduced, when, and to whom, is usually at the discretion of the provider. If a person is diagnosed with type 2 diabetes, initial management is education for lifestyle change with or without an oral hypoglycaemic. As the disease progresses, oral medications are added in a stepwise fashion and eventually insulin may be introduced. Education, considered the cornerstone of diabetes management, consists of teaching patients the reasons why they should follow the management regime that has been chosen for them.

So why is there this push for providers to follow guidelines and protocols? In the first of a four-part series, the US Institute of Medicine[2] (now the Health and Medicine Division of the National Academies of Sciences, Engineering, and Medicine) proposes five potential benefits to clinical guidelines: they ensure evidence-based practice, improve outcomes, minimise mistakes, minimise waste and cut costs. In other words, the argument runs, following protocols allows clinicians to provide the very best, safest, most efficient and most cost-effective care to all patients at all times. But is this in fact the case? And are we doing the right thing? Should we be approaching every patient with diabetes with the same management plan? Certainly, despite these alleged benefits of a standardised approach, we are not doing very well. We have escalating medical costs, escalating incidence of complications, escalating societal costs for income support and disability, poor patient compliance, poor provider compliance, poor outcomes and poor patient satisfaction.[1,3] Indeed, in their series of articles, the Institute of Medicine is quick to point out that, while protocols and guidelines purport to have potential benefits, these benefits come with some significant limitations as well as some possible harms.

No one would question the success of the conventional model of disease management for acute episodic care. In fact, one of the major contributing factors to the epidemic of chronic disease has been the success of acute disease management. Despite its success, however, the acute disease management model has been criticised for its oversimplification of illness.[4,5] Guidelines such as those mentioned above make two assumptions: that disease pathology and progression is stereotypic from one case to the next, and that there is only one correct way to treat a disease. As Engel wrote in 1977, the conventional acute care model

"...assumes disease to be fully accounted for by deviations from the norm of measurable biological (somatic) variables. It leaves no room within its framework for the social, psychological and behavioural dimensions of illness. The biomedical model not only requires that disease be dealt with as an entity independent of social behaviour, it also demands that behavioural aberrations be explained on the basis of disordered somatic (biochemical or neurophysiological) processes".[6]

The very nature of acute disease, where the underlying cause is generally one pathology easily targeted by one treatment and with a rapid road to complete recovery, is forgiving of such 'simplifications', as witnessed by the success of the conventional disease management model. Unfortunately, as will be outlined below, the very nature of chronic disease not only highlights the limitations of these 'simplifications', but exposes them for what they really are – significant barriers to care.

Chronic disease is more complex than acute disease, both medically and psychosocially: there is usually more than one pathophysiologic mechanism underlying the disease, there are often multiple comorbidities needing medical management, and the disease is not being managed within a controlled environment such as a hospital but at home under the care of the patient. In an attempt to better address these medical and psychosocial complexities, guidelines began to recommend that care for diabetes be provided by multidisciplinary teams.[7-10] How different members of a multidisciplinary team interact with each other and the patient has been the subject of much research and has resulted in a number of models of care being advocated.[11-14]

Unfortunately, regardless of the model of care, this multidisciplinary approach has not been particularly successful, as evidenced by continuing poor health outcomes. Perhaps this should not come as a surprise. After all, these multidisciplinary teams are simply variations of the provider-centric, 'one size fits all' approach, with the doctor dictating disease management according to protocol, the dietician instructing the patient on what they can and cannot eat, nurse educators and/or group education sessions instructing patients on how to comply with the recommended management – and when the patient is 'non-compliant', the psychologist attempts to alleviate the burden of these enforced lifestyle changes. The patient is still very much the passive recipient of a prescribed management regime that is based on a stereotypic disease pathology and leaves little room for individual needs or preferences. As appropriately articulated by the Institute of Medicine, simply "adding greater expectations on simple solutions to systems designed for a different set of healthcare problems is unlikely to be successful. The system must change."[2]

Recognising the significant influence psychosocial factors have on disease management, and stimulated by studies demonstrating the effectiveness of self-management, new models of care are shifting from treatment that is done to passive recipients by medical experts to treatment that is planned collaboratively with patients.[14] Key influences behind this shift have been the Chronic Care Model[16] and the Institute of Medicine report, *Crossing the Quality Chasm*.[2] Both place the provision of patient-centred care at the heart of their models of care.

Patient-centred clinical medicine is a *formal theoretical framework*[17] that recognises the uniqueness of an individual's disease, the uniqueness of their life commitments, their leisure activities as well as the uniqueness of their personal experience of the disease due to culture, beliefs and previous experience with the disease. Patient-centred care is "respectful of and responsive to individual patient preferences, needs and values…ensuring that patient values guide all clinical decisions".[3] Thus, patient-centred care recognises that the patient is the real expert in the room when it comes to choosing which management regime will work best for them and, as such, their illness cannot be adequately managed without their acquiring a full understanding of their disease and all current management options.[15]

The term 'patient-centred medicine' was first introduced 50 years ago by Balint and his colleagues.[17] However, it was not until the mid-1980s that the patient-centred clinical method as we understand it today was first conceptualised and used in research and education.[18] In 1995, *Patient-Centered Medicine: Transforming the Clinical Method* by Stewart et al. placed this model of care at the epicentre of clinical practice internationally.[17] Patient-centred care has proven to be cost-effective with a positive impact on health outcomes and healthcare utilisation,[19,20] and in 2001 the Institute of Medicine included it as one of the six core attributes necessary for a quality healthcare system.[3] By 2012 the American Diabetes Association recognised "individualization of treatment [as] the cornerstone of success",[21] and since then has continued to emphasise the need for a patient-centred approach in all subsequent publications on the standards of diabetes care.

Unfortunately, as the patient-centred clinical method has become more mainstream, the term has become overused, bandied about without a true understanding of what this model of care really entails. Disappointingly, the phrase is often misinterpreted or misunderstood to mean care that simply focuses on the patient. However, this is absolutely what it is not. As emphasised by Churchill, providers must "embark upon therapeutic encounters with patients … not by making the relationship with their patients central, but by making their patients and their patients' needs central".[22]

To ensure care is truly patient-centred, several clinical requisites need to be included within every patient–provider interaction: establishing a working relationship, finding a common language, understanding the patient, acknowledging the patient as the expert, finding common ground and empowering the patient. On the face of it, these seem relatively straightforward, simple principles to follow. However, after reviewing the following descriptions of each requisite, one will realise that most clinical encounters do not adhere to many of these principles. It will also become obvious that for these requisites to be successfully implemented, it is not the current 'system of care' that needs to change, but the behaviour of the provider that must change.

ESTABLISH A WORKING RELATIONSHIP

For the vast majority, visits to a healthcare provider are about addressing a symptom or other health-related concern with an acute onset, such as a fever or sore ear. During these visits the expectation, on the part of both the provider and the patient, is that the provider as expert will establish a diagnosis and make management recommendations which the patient will then follow if they wish to get better. This means that any patient arriving at any healthcare appointment, regardless of the issue at hand, generally expects to be a passive recipient of care. Clearly, this is the antithesis to a patient-centred approach, where the provider steps back to the role of educator, wanting the patient, as expert, to actively participate in and guide all disease management decisions. Thus, for patient-centred care to be successful, it is imperative that this reversal of roles be openly established right from the start. The provider must acknowledge the patient as the expert and do it in such a way that the patient accepts this role and willingly steps up to be an active participant.

This role reversal is not difficult to achieve. Indeed, once it is explained, patients are usually eager to adopt their new role. Below is the conversation I have with each patient at the beginning of their first visit.

Before we start talking about your diabetes, I would like to point out to you that we approach things a little differently from what you have possibly experienced in the past. I want you to take a minute to think back to when you were first diagnosed with diabetes. I imagine that it went something like this: "Now that you have diabetes we need you take these pills. It would also be good to lose some weight and exercise 20 minutes of every day. You will need to stop eating some of your favourite foods, and you need to quit smoking…." In other words, we were telling you what to do with the expectation that you should rearrange your life so that it fits into the management of your diabetes.

Well, we take a different approach here. We are very lucky these days, we have many options to choose from when it comes to managing diabetes. I would like to present all these options to you so that you can then pick and choose which management options you feel will work best for you. For example, perhaps you would like to eat chocolate every night before bed; in which case, I can show you a number of management options that would allow you to have the chocolate and have a normal blood sugar after the chocolate. In other words, you can choose management options so that your diabetes management fits into your life.

Does this sound like something that you would like to try?

Because we are looking to fit diabetes management into your life, I consider you to be the expert when it comes to choosing your management regime. Afterall, I have never met you before; I have no understanding of your life and what is important to you. Indeed, only you truly understand the complexities and demands of your daily life and know your wishes, desires and beliefs; as such, it is you who are the expert when it comes to making decisions around your disease management. My role is simply to provide you with information so that you can make well-informed decisions.

So, as you are the expert in the room, I am going to be looking to you for decision-making. I am simply here to support you with information so that you can be comfortable with your decisions.

Are you ok with this plan?

FIND A COMMON LANGUAGE

If a person is to make sound decisions around their diabetes management, then that person must be fully informed. This means education must be detailed and disease-specific so that each patient fully understands not just disease pathology, but *their* disease pathology; they need to know of all the available treatment options, how they work, the advantages and disadvantages of each, and they need to understand the long-term health consequences of different management choices. Obviously, all information provided should be evidence-based.

To successfully transfer all this information, a 'common language' must be established. This means finding simple but comprehensive ways to translate medical terminology into a language that is understandable to the patient. This does not mean simplifying the physiology and pharmacology in an attempt to make it understandable; it means *simplifying the language to ensure that ALL the complexities of the physiology and pharmacology will be understood.*

Should any detail be left out, the patient will no longer be in a position to make fully informed decisions. This automatically places the provider back in the 'expert' role, instinctively suggesting management recommendations, and 'education' reverts to coercing the patient into changing their behaviour to fit a set of provider-chosen rules ("you should eat these foods, take these pills") and "promoting self-care behaviours is reduced to simply finding ways to educate and motivate people sufficiently so that they will pursue the [expert-chosen] course of action."[23]

There are many ways to establish a common language, and each provider is encouraged to find the approach that works best for them. Our clinic uses a simple drawing (see Patient Handout 1). Details around normal glucose metabolism, the pathophysiology of diabetes and medications are added to the picture in front of the patient as the explanations unfold. How the information is presented and in what order is dependent on the educational level of the patient, on the questions they ask, on the type of diabetes they have, and so on. In the end, each patient may end up with a slightly different looking picture (Figure 11.1), but each will have received the same information.

This same basic drawing has purposely been used throughout this manual (e.g. Figure 1.2) to support the discussions on the pathophysiology of diabetes, medications and insulin use. The goal was to demonstrate how complex and comprehensive medical knowledge can be communicated through the use of simple drawings and language. Other examples of establishing a 'common language' can be found in Chapter 9, Lifestyle Management, and Chapter 10, Cardiovascular Risk Management.

UNDERSTAND THE PATIENT

Each person has their own unique set of understandings, life experiences and personal and cultural belief systems which inextricably contribute to self-management decision-making. Indeed, providers are only too familiar with patients who "love to interpret, evaluate and react to doctors' recommendations based on their personal experience of their illness in the context of their

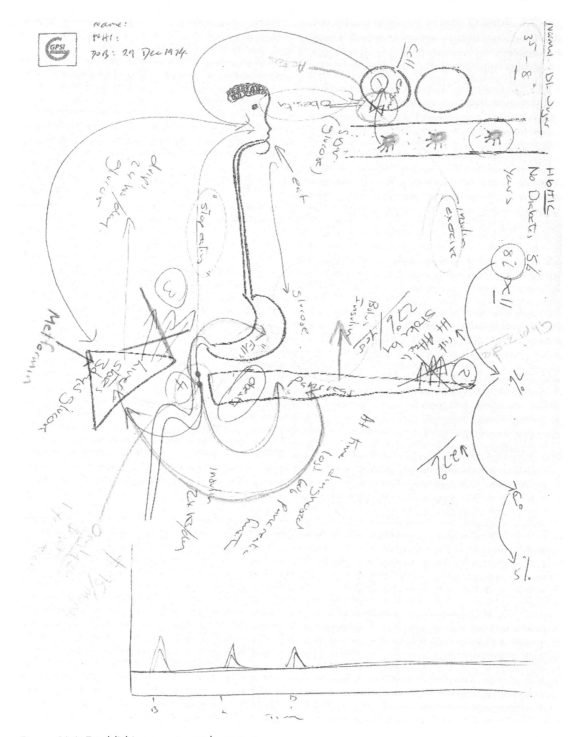

Figure 11.1 Establishing a common language.

lives", resulting in patient management decisions and behaviours that do not coincide with those of the clinician.[24] However, from a patient-centred perspective, this 'non-adherent', 'difficult' or 'non-compliant' patient is seen as a person making the best decisions they can, using the knowledge they have, to adapt a prescribed management regime to fit their understandings, life's demands and expectations. From a patient-centred perspective, a 'non-compliant' patient is not seen as a patient failing to comply with treatment, but an indication of failure on the part of the provider to adequately understand what factors are contributing to the patient's decision-making.

To illustrate this point, consider how very different the impact of being newly diagnosed with diabetes could be from one person to the next. For someone who has never met anyone with diabetes, being given a new diagnosis may be relatively inconsequential due to their lack of knowledge or understanding of diabetes. However, for someone who is caring for a family member with bilateral lower extremity amputations, blindness and on renal dialysis, the impact of receiving a new diagnosis will likely be considerable. Furthermore, how each person emotionally and intellectually interprets their life experiences will also influence how they choose to care for their diabetes; both may choose to do nothing (one out of ignorance, the other out of hopelessness), or both may choose to do everything (the first because they fear the unknown, the second because of a true understanding of the consequences of poor management).

Thus, within the patient-centred paradigm, if a patient's management decisions and behaviours do not coincide with those of the provider, the provider must not label the patient as 'non-compliant'. Rather, they must recognise that the patient's behaviour is the result of complex decision-making (conscious or subconscious), facilitated or hindered by many factors,[25] and *it is the responsibility of the provider* to systematically explore their patient's experiences and understandings so they can identify the factors that are contributing to the patient's behaviours – i.e. the provider must seek to 'understand the patient'. Only when the provider understands what is contributing to a patient's decision-making or behaviour can appropriate support and education be provided – tailored to fill gaps in the patient's knowledge and remove myths and misinformation,

ultimately allowing the patient to make sound decisions.

ACKNOWLEDGE THE PATIENT AS THE EXPERT

By recognising the patient as the expert, the provider must accept the patient's management choices as those that are most likely to succeed for that patient. The provider must also accept the possibility that a patient may make very different management choices from what the provider might have made.

Of course, there is the possibility that the decisions made by the patient could be unsound, medically. Logically, this should not happen if the patient is fully informed. However, should this happen, it is likely due to a gap in the patient's knowledge or a misunderstanding. So, when a patient is making choices that the provider regards as inappropriate, it is important go back and take the time to understand where the patient is coming from and ensure that there are no misunderstandings or gaps in their knowledge.

FIND COMMON GROUND

This is probably the hardest concept of patient-centred care to convey – and the hardest patient-centred skill to master.

The tendency for many providers, when trying to motivate a patient to do better with their diabetes self-management, is to impose external motivators – "If you don't take your pills then you are going to lose your eye sight", or, "Wouldn't you like to be around to see your grandchildren grow up?" However, change in human behaviour only occurs when people are intrinsically motivated; having someone or something imposing an external motivator does not produce long-term behavioural changes.[26] This understanding sits at the very core of the patient-centred model of care, and to 'find common ground' is to find the patient's internal motivator (which may or may not have anything to do with diabetes) that will align their behaviour with the provider's desired outcome (e.g. increased regularity of blood glucose testing, lowering of HbA_{1c}).

For the most part, finding a patient's internal motivator is relatively straightforward. Providing education so they become fully informed is all that is needed; explaining HbA$_{1c}$ and how it predicts their personal risk of diabetes-related complications works extremely well (see explanation, Chapter 10, Cardiovascular Risk Management).

However, in other cases, finding common ground can be difficult and will require the provider to take the time to explore and understand the patient's values, beliefs, motivations and life commitments, so that reasons for improving their diabetes management can be presented (either surreptitiously or blatantly) as a means of improving some aspect of their life that is important to them.[27-29] Common ground with a young man entering into a serious relationship may be his wish to restore/maintain erectile function; or with a drummer in a band, as in the case below, it may be his desire to perfect his fine motor coordination.

CASE EXAMPLE

A young man with type 1 diabetes rarely checked his blood sugars. He "could not be bothered"; he was too busy. Subsequent conversation revealed that life was good; he was the drummer in a successful band and he was spending every spare moment practising. He loved to practise especially on the days when his timing was good. However, he would get a bit frustrated on the days when his timing was off. After explaining to the young man that coordination and reaction time deteriorate when blood sugars are outside normal range, the provider suggested he might want to go away and see if there was any correlation between his blood sugars and his 'off' days. He discovered, of course, that on the days that his timing was off, his blood sugars were very high. Not surprisingly, this young man now checks his blood sugars and gives insulin prior to each practise session and gig.

In his case, 'finding common ground' meant aligning his desire to improve timing and coordination with the provider's goal of increasing the frequency of blood glucose checks and insulin delivery.

EMPOWER THE PATIENT

If a patient has participated in their choice of management, and common ground (self-motivation) has been established, then little support is needed to keep the patient following their chosen self-management regime. However, diabetes is a progressive disease requiring ongoing monitoring and adjustment of lifestyle choices, medications and insulin doses. As people with diabetes are responsible for their day-to-day management, providing more than 90% of their own care,[30] no one is in a better position than themselves to monitor their diabetes and make adjustments to their management regime. Thus, the final step towards a fully independent self-managing patient is to provide each patient with a set of skills for 'focused' self-monitoring. Which set of skills is taught and which type of strategy is taken will be unique to each patient depending on what management choices they have made, what is important to them and what their physical and/or intellectual abilities are. Specifics as to how to do this safely are provided in the next chapter, Chapter 12, Empowering the Patient for Lifelong Self-Management.

Sceptics have voiced a number of concerns about the patient-centred model of care. Some believe that providing patient-centred care will take more time;[17,30] others complain that it focuses "primarily on the patient's psychosocial issues rather than their disease".[17] However, research has shown that patient-centred consultations do not take longer.[31,32] Indeed, visits where providers respond to patients' psychosocial and/or emotional concerns are shorter than visits in which providers adhere to their own agenda.[17] Patient-centred visits are also associated with greater patient satisfaction,[33-37] better patient adherence to chosen management plans,[37,38] better self-reported health[20] and improved clinical outcomes.[31,39]

However, as noted earlier, for clinicians to transition to this new consultant/partnership role, a significant change in skills and mindset is needed.[40] Indeed, as emphasised by Stewart et al.,

"it is important not to underestimate the magnitude of the changes implied by the transformation of the patient-centred clinical method. It is not simply a matter of learning some new techniques, though that is part of it. Nor is it only a question of adding courses in interviewing and behavioural science to the curriculum. The *change goes much deeper than that. It requires nothing less than a change in what it means to be a physician, a different way of thinking about health and disease....*[17]

SUMMARY

- The current model of healthcare has evolved to manage acute episodic illness and is ill-suited to approaching the complexities of chronic disease.
- Patient-centred clinical medicine is a formal theoretical framework that recognises the uniqueness of an individual's disease, the uniqueness of their life's commitments and leisure activities, and the uniqueness of their personal experience of the disease due to culture, beliefs and previous experience with the disease.
- Patient-centred medicine requires a reversal of roles with the patient regarded as the expert when it comes to choosing their diabetes management regime; the provider is an educator whose goal is to ensure the patient is well informed.
- To ensure care is truly patient-centred, several clinical requisites must be included within every patient–provider interaction: establishing a working relationship, finding a common language, understanding the patient, accepting the patient as the expert, finding common ground and empowering the patient.
- For clinicians to transition to providing patient-centred care, a significant change in skills and mindset is needed. It is not the current 'system of care' that needs to change, but the behaviour of the provider.

REFERENCES

1. Fisher L, Glasgow RE. A call for more effectively integrating behavioural and social science principles into comprehensive diabetes care. Diabetes Care. 2007; 30:2746–2749

2. Institute of Medicine. Crossing the quality chasm: a new health system for the 21st century. National Academy Press, Washington DC, 2001
3. Kahn R, Anderson JE. Improving diabetes care: the model of health care reform. Diabetes Care. 2009;32:1115–1118
4. Odgarrd CE. Dear Doctor – a personal letter to a physician. The Henry J Kaiser Family Foundation, Menlo Park, CA, 1986
5. White KL. The task of medicine: dialogue at Wickenburg. The Henry J Kaiser Family Foundation, Menlo Park CA, 1988
6. Engel GL. The need for a new medical model: a challenge for biomedicine. Science. 1977;196(4286):535–544
7. American Diabetes Association. Standards of medical care for patients with diabetes mellitus. Diabetes Care. 1989;12:365–36
8. Bodenheimer T. Coordinating care: a perilous journey through the health care system. N Engl J Med. 2008;358:1064–1071
9. Kellerman R, Kirk L. Principles of the patient centered medical home. Am Fam Physician. 2007;76:774–775
10. Marshall SM. Intensive diabetes management for high-risk patients: how best to deliver? Diabetes Care. 2009;32:1132–1133
11. Coleman K, Austin BT, Brach C, Wagner EH. Evidence on the chronic care model in the new millennium. Health Aff. 2009;28:75–85
12. McLean DL, McAlister FA, Johnson JA, et al. A randomized trial of the effect of community pharmacist and nurse care on improving blood pressure management in patients with diabetes mellitus. Arch Intern Med. 2008;168:2355–2361
13. Shojania KG, Ranji SR, McDonald KM, et al. Effects of quality improvement strategies for type 2 diabetes on glycemic control. JAMA. 2006;296:427–440
14. Davidson MB. How our medical care system fails people with diabetes: lack of timely, appropriate clinical decisions. Diabetes Care. 2009;32:370–372
15. Glasgow RE, Peeples M, Skovlund SE. Where is the patient in diabetes performance measures? The case for including patient-centered and self-management measures. Diabetes Care. 2008;31:1046–1050
16. Bodenheimer TS, Wagner EH, Grumbach K. Improving primary care for patients with chronic illness. JAMA. 2002;288:1775–1779
17. Stewart M, Brown JB, Weston WW, et al. Patient-centered medicine. Transforming the

clinical method, 2nd ed. Radcliffe Medical Press, Oxford UK, 2003

18. Brown JB, Stewart MA, McCracken EC, et al. Patient-centered clinical method II. Definition and application. Fam Pract. 1986;3:75–79

19. Little P, Everitt H, Williamson I, et al. Observational study of effect of patient centredness and positive approach on outcomes of general practice consultations. BMJ. 2001;323:908–911

20. Stewart M, Brown JB, Donner A, et al. The impact of patient-centred care on outcomes. J Fam Pract. 2000;49:796–804

21. Inzucchi SE, Bergenstal RM, Buse JB, et al. Management of hyperglycemia in type 2 diabetes: a patient-centered approach. Position statement of the American Diabetes Association and the European Association of the Study of Diabetes. Diabetes Care. 2012;35:1364–1379

22. Churchill LR. 'Damaged humanity': the call for a patient-centered medical ethic in the managed care era. Theor Med. 1997;18:113–126

23. Hunt LM, Arar NH. An analytical framework for contrasting patient and provider views of the process of chronic disease management. Med Anthropol Q. 2001;15:347–67.

24. Heisler M, Resnicow K. Helping patients make and sustain healthy changes: a brief introduction to motivational interviewing in clinical diabetes care. Clin Diabetes. 2008;26:161–165

25. Bauman L. A patient-centered approach to adherence: risks of non-adherence. In Dortar D (ed) Promoting adherence to medical treatment in chronic childhood illness. L Earlbaum Associates Ltd, Mahwah USA, 2000, p 520.

26. Nelson JB. A motivational challenge: blending practice with theory. AADE Pract. March 2014:42–43

27. Norris SL, Engelgau MM, Narayan KM. Effectiveness of self-management training in type 2 diabetes: a systematic review of randomized controlled trials. Diabetes Care. 2001;24:561–587

28. Bodenheimer T, Lorig K, Holman H, Grumbach K. Patient self-management of chronic disease in primary care. JAMA. 2002;288:2469–2475

29. Holman H, Lorig K. Patients as partners in managing chronic disease: partnership is a prerequisite for effective and efficient healthcare. BMJ. 2000;320:526–527.

30. Anderson RM, Patrias R. Getting out ahead: the Diabetes Concerns Assessment Form. Clin Diabetes. 2007;25(4):141–143

31. Greenfield S, Kaplan S, Ware JE Jr. Patients' participation in medical care: effects on blood sugar and quality of life in diabetes. J Gen Intern Med. 1988;3:448–457

32. Henbest RJ, Fehresen GS. Patient-centredness: is it applicable outside the West? Its measurement and effect on outcomes. Fam Pract. 1992;9:311–317

33. Dietrich AJ, Marton KI. Does continuous care from a physician make a difference? J Fam Pract. 1982;15:929–937

34. Hall JA, Dornan MC. Meta-analysis of satisfaction with medical care: description of research domain and analysis of overall satisfaction levels. Soc Sci Med. 1988;27:637–644

35. Hall JA, Dornan MC. What patients like about their medical care and how often they are asked: a meta-analysis of the satisfaction literature. Soc Sci Med. 1988;27:635–639

36. Linn MW, Linn BS, Stein SR. Satisfaction with ambulatory care and compliance in older patients. Med Care. 1982;20:606–614

37. Stewart M, Brown JB, Boon H, et al. Evidence on patient–doctor communication. Cancer Prev Control. 1999;3:25–30

38. Golin CE, DiMatteo MR, Gelberg L. The role of patient participation in the doctor visit. Implications for adherence to diabetes care. Diabetes Care. 1996;19:1153–1164

39. Kaplan SH, Greenfield S, Ware JE. Assessing the effects of physician–patient interactions on the outcomes of chronic disease. Med Care. 1989;27(3suppl):S110–127

40. O'Donnell M, Parker G, Proberts M, et al. A study of client-focused case management and consumer advocacy: the community and consumer service project. Aust N Z J Psychiatry. 1999;33:684–693

12

Empowering the patient for lifelong self-management

Typically, when a patient has been actively involved in the decision-making for their diabetes management, they have a vested interest in their ongoing self-management and, if common ground has been established, little support is needed to keep the patient following their chosen management regime. However, diabetes is a progressive disease and requires ongoing monitoring and adjustment of lifestyle choices, medications and insulin doses. Changes in other medical and/or psychosocial conditions can also occur, possibly even rearranging a person's priorities and beliefs so that the current management regime is no longer a good fit. So, what is currently working for a person's diabetes management will likely not continue to do so.

Thus, to support long-term diabetes control, the final task of a patient-centred provider is to empower the patient with the skills necessary for monitoring deterioration in blood sugar control and/or changes in their own self-management behaviours; and if changes are noted, patients should be provided with the skills to address the changes so they can continue to stay on course.

Empowering a patient for ongoing self-management is not difficult. The biggest barrier is usually the provider struggling to give up a position of control. To be successful, three principles need to be followed: ensure there is always opportunity for ongoing education; put 'supports' and 'safety nets' in place, so that both the patient and the provider know the patient is safe; and, finally, hand over the controls.

PROVIDE OPPORTUNITY FOR ONGOING EDUCATION

Accurate and detailed knowledge is the most powerful way to empower a patient to successfully manage their diabetes. Throughout this manual considerable time has been spent either using or presenting different ways that knowledge and understanding can be transferred to patients. But it is important that this imparting of knowledge is ongoing, occurring with every patient interaction, so that over time each patient will become increasingly more independent with their self-management.

This means that every patient–provider interaction, whether in person, by telephone or over the internet, should be regarded as a 'teachable moment': a golden opportunity to further educate and upskill the patient. This can only be achieved by the provider making a subtle but important shift in their behaviour; the provider must shift the focus of every patient interaction from the task of managing the disease of diabetes to the task of educating the patient, so that the patient is the one making well-informed decisions on how they will manage their disease. Thus, the ever-present reviewing of blood tests for the fine-tuning of medical management is no longer the provider's primary purpose in a diabetes appointment – the primary purpose is to use the blood test results as the catalyst for educating and upskilling the patient.

Keep in mind that incorrect or lack of knowledge is just as influential on behaviour as correct knowledge. This means that if a person presents to their appointment not doing well, it is important to go back to the basics: do not hesitate to pull out the picture, re-establish a common language, review underlying pathophysiology and the mechanisms of medications, making sure there are no gaps in the patient's knowledge and that the information is not being reinterpreted inappropriately. It is also important to take the time to once again 'understand the patient', as it is very possible that some new idea or experienced event has altered how they are thinking about their diabetes – as in the case presented below.

CASE EXAMPLE

Maria is a 17 year old with type 1 diabetes. She has always had a very good understanding of her diabetes and how to manage it with adjustments to insulin doses for food and blood sugars. However, over the past couple of months, the frequency of her blood sugar checks has dropped off and she presents with a worsening HbA$_{1c}$.

On drawing attention to the sporadic blood sugar checks, Maria states that she just doesn't seem to remember to do them anymore; she is too busy. Clearly, Maria's mum has also noticed the lack of blood sugar checks as Maria happens to mention that her mother is driving her mad, constantly on her back reminding her to check.

It is pointed out to Maria that even when mum has reminded her, the checks don't seem to be happening, suggesting that not remembering is not the sole reason for her lack of blood glucose checks. Maria acknowledges this and initially is not able to provide a reason as to why she is not checking when her mother reminds her. All that she knows is that she no longer wants to know what the blood sugar reading might be.

When asked why she no longer wants to know what her blood sugar reading is, Maria bursts into tears; she states that she has become too scared to check her blood sugars because she is worried that if her

blood sugars are really high, she is going to instantly drop dead. She would just rather not know. With a little more probing, we find out that her mother has been repeatedly reminding Maria that "you know if you have high sugars – you are going to die". After redirecting Maria's inappropriate belief (and her mother's behaviours), Maria was very quickly back on track.

ENSURE SUPPORT AND SAFETY NETS ARE IN PLACE – FOR BOTH PATIENT AND PROVIDER

While a provider offering patient-centred care is placing the patient in the 'expert' role, this does not necessarily mean the patient is confident in their ability to fulfil this role; nor does it mean the provider will have confidence in the patient's ability to fulfil the role. This will be especially true at the beginning of the working relationship. But it will also be true any time a new skill is being taught. Thus, it is important to put good supports in place both for the patient and the provider. If good supports are not in place, the patient will not become a confident self-manager and the provider will not be willing to 'cut the apron strings', diminishing the chances that the patient will progress to managing their diabetes independently.

The analogy of learning to ride a bike fits well here. When a child is learning to ride, most parents will begin by providing significant support: hold the bike to help with balance, run alongside, offer tips on how to steer and how to peddle. For the parent, this means they can be confident that the child will not fall and hurt themselves. For the child, it means they feel safe, knowing that they will not fall. With emotions such as fear removed, the child can focus on acquiring the skills of how to ride; they might even push their boundaries, take a few risks and be able to learn from any mistakes, safely. As the child's skill level improves and their confidence builds, the parent supports the bike less and less. But should the parent pull the support away too quickly, the child may fall and lose confidence; progress in learning will take a step backwards, and supports will need to be re-established until the child's and the parent's confidence has returned.

Obviously, some children will require more support than others and some will take longer to learn the skills needed. Furthermore, if supports are individualised, a child with a learning disability, coordination issue, or even a physical disability can also be given the opportunity to learn to ride a bike. The take-home message is that, as long as supports are tailored to the individual, any child can learn to ride a bike. How this analogy translates into teaching the skills of diabetes self-management is obvious: if the right supports are put in place *all* people with diabetes can self-manage their diabetes.

Remember also that, if care is to be truly patient-centred, every patient should be provided with information about all the available management options, regardless of whether the provider believes the management option is appropriate or within the patient's budget and/or physical abilities. It is up to the patient to decide whether or not they believe there are limitations. Unfortunately, because of preconceived ideas about patients' abilities (financial, physical or intellectual), providers sometimes choose to withhold information and/or teaching of skills. I have seen providers withhold initiation of insulin for a person with an unsteady hand secondary to Parkinson's disease, or not teach a flexible insulin regime to a high school dropout. Yet both of these patients had jobs, drove cars and could manage a TV remote control – all great measures of having sufficient problem-solving capabilities and coordination to master desirable skills. It is my experience that taking time to explore apparent barriers will almost always result in a solution being found, while withholding information and/or support risks introducing inequalities in diabetes care. Indeed, it has been well established that the stereotypic assumptions of providers often result in different care for minority patient groups.[1] Furthermore, as soon as a provider begins to be selective about which knowledge or skill to include in their teachings, the patient's ability to make fully informed choices about their own care is jeopardised. In fact, a patient-centred purist would consider a patient's inability to master self-management as a reflection of incomplete or inappropriate education and support being put in place by the provider.

The number and types of support that can be put in place are infinite and clearly depend on what physical, emotional and intellectual limitations one is faced with. Examples of supports would include:

- Offering frequent and/or extended visits – especially for those with English as a second language.
- Inviting family members to attend appointments so that they can learn new skills (e.g. carbohydrate counting) alongside the patient and provide support at home.
- Offering a telephone contact service for those who are learning to adjust insulin doses; encouraging them to call when they are struggling with a dose calculation.
- Giving patients 'permission' to call the office for appointments when things are not going well. Many patients feel guilty about 'bothering' the doctor.
- Tailoring equipment to a patient's needs, e.g. talking blood glucose meters for the visually impaired, magnifiers for syringes, wrap tape around the bolus insulin pen for tactile labelling for a visually impaired person.
- For a person with a physical or intellectual disability that limits their ability to manage insulin syringes, having a family member, pharmacist or support person draw up a week's supply of fixed insulin doses in syringes and store these in the fridge.
- Providing written instructions to support any teaching such as a person's correction factor, i.e. sliding scale (see Patient Handouts 7 and 8).

Once appropriate supports have been put in place, it is equally important to put 'safety nets' in place. These minimise the risk of injury. They also permit the patient to learn confidently and the provider to feel comfortable that the patient is not going to get into difficulty. Once again, the analogy of a child learning to ride a bike is useful. A 'safety net' in this scenario could be the setting of strict parameters around where the child is permitted to ride (e.g. driveway versus road) or insisting that a helmet be worn at all times.

Once again, the type of 'safety net' being put in place will very much depend on individual patient needs. Examples are:

- If the provider and/or the patient is not confident about the patient's ability to do calculations correctly while learning carbohydrate counting, decrease the basal insulin dose. This allows room for the patient to make a mistake without the risk of a major hypoglycaemic episode.

- When the patient is learning a correction factor, keep the target blood glucose on the high side, i.e. correct to 10 mmol/L (180 mg/dL) – not to 5 mmol/L (90 mg/dL).
- Establish a set of call parameters and have the patient enter into a 'contract' with the provider to call if the parameters are met, e.g. "If you are getting blood sugars less than 4 mmol/L (or 70 mg/dL) more than five times a week, call this number …."

Contracting with a patient not only provides a level of comfort around patient safety but also provides reassurance as to whether the patient is truly committed to self-management. A patient not following through with a contractual agreement is a great indication that something has been missed in the process of establishing an empowered patient; perhaps there is a gap or misunderstanding in their knowledge, or common ground has not been successfully established. When this happens, one needs to go right back to the basics to determine what is missing.

CASE EXAMPLE

So, John, now that you have learnt how to carbohydrate count, do you think you can try this at home? I think you will do great.

But let's figure out some follow-up.

I have just calculated your carb ratio based on a formula and your current insulin doses. I am sure that the ratio I've calculated is pretty close to where it should be, but it may need a little fine-tuning. So, how do you feel about touching base with me tomorrow at 5 p.m. with a phone call, just so I can see how it's working?

Obviously, call me sooner if things are not going well for you – indeed, should you get a blood sugar less than 3.0 mmol/mol (55 mg/dL), I would really like you to call, as clearly an adjustment needs to be made.

Are you OK with calling me?

HAND OVER THE CONTROLS

For the most part, monitoring for disease progression is seen as the provider's responsibility. To assist providers with this task, most clinics have introduced electronic medical record systems with clinical alerts to ensure patients are recalled for blood tests and appointments on a regular basis. This has placed a significant burden on the current workforce. Indeed, workforce limitation secondary to the demands of chronic disease management is considered one of the major challenges for the provision of healthcare today.[2]

However, if the expectation of monitoring and managing diabetes (or any other condition for that matter) is shifted from the provider to the person with diabetes, this would go a long way to alleviating this burden. In fact, a person who is well informed and managing their diabetes on a day-to-day basis is going to be in a far better position to monitor and make timely management changes than a provider who only interacts with that patient periodically.

For a person who has been at the receiving end of patient-centred care, little more in the way of education is needed to ensure they understand how to monitor for disease deterioration, how to make changes to their own medical management and how and when to ask for help if they find themselves struggling with management decisions. Thus, every patient-centred care provider should strive to transfer all their knowledge to each patient with the idealistic intention of doing themselves out of business; our role should simply be to educate and support only when needed. So, once the patient has acquired a sound knowledge base around day-to-day management of their diabetes and supports and safety nets have been put in place, it is time to hand over the controls.

Empowering a patient for long-term self-management means providing each patient with a set of instructions around what signals disease deterioration, how to monitor for it and what to do if deterioration is noted. Once again, as everyone's diabetes management is different, as their social, intellectual and physical abilities are different, these instructions must be tailored to each individual. However, with every patient, key elements that should be covered are:

- Ensure the patient understands how the HbA_{1c} and blood glucose checks contribute different information with regard to how their diabetes is doing. Remind the patient that the benchmark for diabetes management is HbA_{1c} (not blood sugars) as it is the HbA_{1c} that is predictive of long-term cardiovascular health. Some patients have a tendency to 'over-control' blood sugars, particularly if they have a high level of self-management skills, so it is important they do not lose sight of the big picture (minimising cardiovascular risk on the basis of HbA_{1c}) when focusing on the minutiae around blood sugar variability. Conversely, it is important that patients understand the need to review blood sugars to rule out hypoglycaemic events and/or widely swinging blood sugars even when HbA_{1c} is at target.
- Ensure the person understands what their target HbA_{1c} is.
- Ensure the patient understands how pre- and postprandial blood sugars reflect different pathologies and what role each of their medications or insulins play in the management of each (see Blood Glucose Management in Chapter 8, Glycaemic Management).
- Provide parameters around blood glucose levels that indicate when a change in management is needed. Review how changes in each of the patient's medications/insulins will selectively alter pre- or post-meal blood sugars. Instructions should be specific to each person's management regime and tailored to each patient's abilities. For example, a patient can be instructed to make changes to their own insulin doses ("increase your Lantus by 10%"), or they can be provided with information on how to contact a provider for assistance with dose changes. Patient Handouts 5 and 6 provide an example of one such set of instructions for a person on a basal insulin.
- *Always* give parameters for when to call for help. If you are expecting a patient to get in contact with a provider, do make sure the arrangements are fail-safe. Also make sure that the patient can access the offered support system (e.g. do they have access to a phone?). Finally, ensure they are comfortable with contacting the clinic. Many patients,

particularly those from the older generation, are reluctant to "bother the doctor".
- As each person's diabetes and diabetes management regime is unique, provide each with their own personal plan for the monitoring of disease progression. For example:
  - For a person on oral medications, monitoring for disease progression can be done by regular HbA_{1c} checks. If the HbA_{1c} is not at target, pre- and postprandial blood glucose checks can be done to assist with management decisions.
  - A person on basal insulin can be instructed to do first morning blood glucose checks for 1 week of every month and, based on their values, alter their basal insulin dose. Clear instructions about when and how to adjust the insulin dose should be given along with clear parameters for calling for further assistance (see Patient Handouts 5 and 6).

Clearly, as a patient's understanding and abilities improve and as management regimes change over time, instructions should be regularly reviewed.

Finally, be realistic, practical and 'user-friendly' with patient self-management expectations:

- Does a person with well-controlled diabetes really need an HbA_{1c} every 3 months?
- Does a person with a new diagnosis of diabetes, well controlled on one oral hypoglycaemic, really need to be monitoring their blood sugars between visits when it is the HbA_{1c} that is going to determine whether something needs to change? Only if the HbA_{1c} is not at target should monitoring of blood sugars be done. Consider having a 'loaner' blood glucose meter with single-use finger-prickers so that such patients do not have to purchase their own.
- Does a person with type 1 diabetes really need to be writing down *all* their blood sugars? More often than not, reviewing the last 3–4 days of blood sugars provides sufficient information for establishing blood glucose patterns. Reviewing pages and pages of numbers rarely offers additional information. A far more practical and user-friendly self-management exercise is to suggest that the patient not write down

their blood sugars, but instead set aside 10 minutes each week (or month) to do a focused review. This can be done by flicking through a meter and writing down the previous 3 days of blood sugars, or by downloading the meter or insulin pump.

- Encourage patients to move away from placing value judgements on blood glucose readings. Blood sugars should not be thought of as 'good' or 'bad'; they should be considered 'as expected' or 'not as expected'. As checking a blood sugar is specifically about making a management decision, then a blood glucose value should simply prompt a series of questions – "is this the number I was expecting?"; if not, then "why is it not the number I was expecting?" This allows a person to learn from their earlier management decisions, to pick up any changes that may be occurring in their management needs, or to raise the suspicion that the insulin pump is not delivering insulin appropriately. The final question should be "what do I need to do with this blood sugar?" By treating each blood glucose check objectively, as a piece of information to be used constructively, a person will continually add to their own understanding of blood sugar management. It also helps them to feel in charge of their diabetes and eliminates the sense of helplessness and guilt that so many people associate with blood sugar checking.
- Ensure each patient understands that diabetes is just one of five clinical parameters contributing to their cardiovascular health, and be sure to provide the same patient-centred approach to support long-term self-management for each of these other parameters.

These skills are not difficult to teach, but for a clinician in a busy practice with limited patient contact time the task can seem somewhat overwhelming. Keep in mind that the up-front demands of educating a patient are short-lived and will ultimately result in better clinical outcomes with reduced utilisation of healthcare services.[3] Remember, too, that providing patient-centred care is not a 'physician-only' skill. Many members of a clinical team can provide the necessary patient support and education; some places have established community 'champions', others provide group education – although (a precautionary note) because education presented in a group setting is 'one size fits all', there is a tendency for group education to lose the individuality and unique approach so essential to the success of patient-centred care.

One last comment: it is essential that positive support be given every step of the way. This means that interactions with a patient must *always* be positive, reassuring, confidence-building, true learning experiences – indeed, a high in the person's day. This includes every interaction with every employee in your office – the front desk staff through to the clinical providers. Unfortunately, some of the biggest barriers to patient self-management are the negative or judgemental messages relayed by the lay public, the media and (sadly) healthcare professionals. Every day, the news is full of depressing statistics about 'diabesity' and the apparent inevitability of associated morbidities and mortalities; it is also one of the few diseases where everyone (family, peers – even strangers) believes that they can be 'helpful' (judgemental?) with their recommendations and 'knowledge'; it is one of the few diseases where healthcare providers openly chastise patients for not 'doing better', often threatening them with comments like "if you don't take these pills, you are going to go blind".

Once again, reflecting on the analogy of the child learning to ride a bike is useful. I do not believe that there would be many parents who would chastise their child each time the child fell off the bike. Should they chastise the child, I suspect most of us would be critical of their attitude. It is much more likely that the parent would come forward, comfort the child, help them back up onto the bike and escalate their support until the child had regained confidence. This is exactly what we should be doing for anyone who is learning to self-manage their diabetes – or any medical condition, for that matter.

SUMMARY

- Empowering a patient for long-term self-management means
  - Making sure every patient–provider interaction is a 'teachable moment'.
  - Putting good supports and safety nets in place so both the patient and provider feel secure and safe.

- Handing over the controls so that each patient can be responsible for their own diabetes monitoring and management.
- A person who is well-informed and managing their diabetes on a day-to-day basis is in a far better position to monitor and make timely management changes than a provider who only interacts with the patient periodically.
- If the right supports are provided, essentially all people with diabetes can self-monitor their own disease and make ongoing management adjustments for long-term diabetes control.
- Be realistic, practical and 'user friendly' with patient self-management expectations.

REFERENCES

1. Smedley BD, Stith AY, Nelson AR (eds). Unequal treatment: confronting racial and ethnic disparities in health care. National Academies Press, Washington DC, 2002
2. Shahady E. The Florida Diabetes Master Clinician Program: facilitating increased quality and significant cost savings for diabetic patients. Clin Diabetes. 2008;26:29–33
3. Stewart M, Brown JB, Donner A, et al. The impact of patient-centred care on outcomes. J Fam Pract. 2000;49:796–804

Index

Note: Page numbers in *italic* denote figures and in **bold** denote tables.

Patient handouts

What is diabetes?

What is HbA$_{1c}$ (mmol/mol)?

What is HbA$_{1c}$ (%)?

HbA$_{1c}$ conversion chart

Monitoring your blood sugars (mmol/L)

Monitoring your blood sugars (mg/dL)

Example: Correction factor (mmol/L)

Example: Correction factor (mg/dL)

Foods

Management of your cardiovascular risk

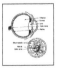
What is a retinal screen?

WHAT IS DIABETES?

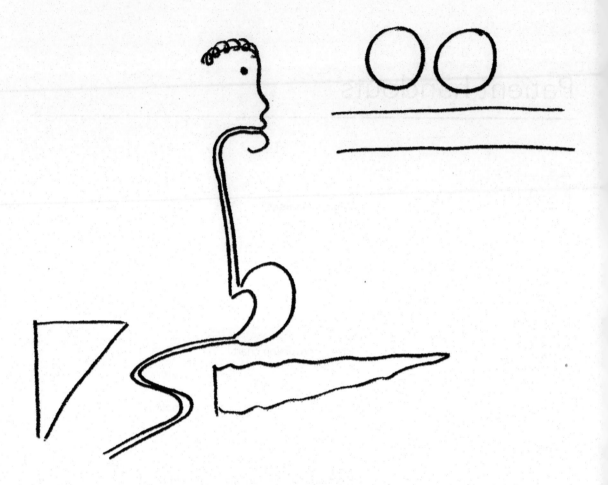

WHAT IS HBA$_{1C}$ (mmol/mol)?

Your HbA$_{1c}$ provides valuable information about your blood glucose control as well as your long-term health.

Glucose travels to all parts of our body within our blood vessels. As it travels, it has a tendency to 'stick' to things such as the insides of the blood vessel walls and to anything else that is travelling within the blood vessels, such as red blood cells. The HbA$_{1c}$ is a measure of how much of the surface of the red blood cell is covered with glucose.

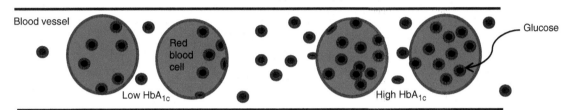

In a person who does not have diabetes, about 5% of the surface of the red blood cell is covered, i.e. HbA$_{1c}$ is 5%. As one can imagine, if blood sugars are high, then a greater percentage of the surface of the red blood cells will be coated with glucose and the reported HbA$_{1c}$ will be higher. These days, HbA$_{1c}$ is no longer reported as a percentage; it is reported in the metric units of mmol/mol (see chart below).

By using a conversion chart such as the one below, the HbA$_{1c}$ can be translated into what your average blood sugar has been over the past 3 months.

What your HbA$_{1c}$ results say about your blood glucose control and your long-term health risk		
HbA$_{1c}$ mmol/mol (%)	Average blood glucose (mmol/L)	Health risk
42 (6%)	7.0	Very low
53 (7%)	8.5	Low
64 (8%)	10.2	Good
75 (9%)	11.8	Medium
86 (10%)	13.3	High
97 (11%)	14.9	Very high
108 (12%)	16.5	Extremely high
119 (13%)	18.1	Extremely high
130 (14%)	19.7	Extremely high

The lifespan of a red blood cell is around 3 months. So, every 3 months there is a complete turnover of your red blood cells. This is why you are sent to the lab for an HbA$_{1c}$ check every 3 months and why the HbA$_{1c}$ reading provides us with your average blood sugar for the past 3 months.

Your HbA$_{1c}$ also provides information around your long-term health. A 10 mmol/mol decrease in your HbA$_{1c}$ will reduce your risk of having a heart attack or stroke by 27% per year and your risk of developing eye or kidney disease by 22% per year.

WHAT IS HBA$_{1C}$ (%)?

Your HbA$_{1c}$ provides valuable information about your blood glucose control as well as your long-term health.

Glucose travels to all parts of our body within our blood vessels. As it travels, it has a tendency to 'stick' to things such as the insides of the blood vessel walls and to anything else that is travelling within the blood vessels, such as red blood cells. The HbA$_{1c}$ is a measure of how much of the surface of the red blood cell is covered with glucose.

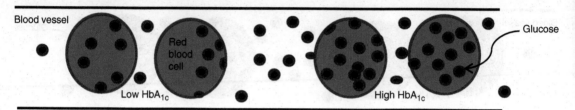

In a person who does not have diabetes, about 5% of the surface of the red blood cell is covered, i.e. HbA$_{1c}$ is 5%. As one can imagine, if blood sugars are high, then a greater percentage of the surface of the red blood cells will be coated with glucose and the reported HbA$_{1c}$ will be higher.

By using a conversion chart such as the one below, the HbA$_{1c}$ can be translated into what your average blood sugar has been over the past 3 months.

What your HbA$_{1c}$ results say about your blood glucose control and your long-term health risk		
HbA$_{1c}$ (%)	Average blood glucose (mg/dL)	Health risk
6	126	Very low
7	154	Low
8	183	Good
9	212	Medium
10	240	High
11	269	Very high
12	298	Extremely high
13	326	Extremely high
14	355	Extremely high

The lifespan of a red blood cell is around 3 months. So, every 3 months there is a complete turnover of your red blood cells. This is why you are sent to the lab for an HbA$_{1c}$ check every 3 months and why the HbA$_{1c}$ reading provides us with your average blood sugar for the past 3 months.

Your HbA$_{1c}$ also provides information around your long-term health. A 1% point decrease in your HbA$_{1c}$ will reduce your risk of having a heart attack or stroke by 27% per year and your risk of developing eye or kidney disease by 22% per year.

HBA$_{1C}$ CONVERSION TABLE

Definitions: old unit (NGSP unit): %; new unit (IFCC unit): mmol/mol
Conversion formulas:
Old = 0.0915 new + 2.15%
New = 10.93 old − 23.5 mmol/mol

HbA$_{1c}$ %	HbA$_{1c}$ mmol/mol	HbA$_{1c}$ %	HbA$_{1c}$ mmol/mol
4.0	20	8.1	65
4.1	21	8.2	66
4.2	22	8.3	67
4.3	23	8.4	68
4.4	25	8.5	69
4.5	26	8.6	70
4.6	27	8.7	72
4.7	28	8.8	73
4.8	29	8.9	74
4.9	30	9.0	75
5.0	31	9.1	76
5.1	32	9.2	77
5.2	33	9.3	78
5.3	34	9.4	79
5.4	36	9.5	80
5.5	37	9.6	81
5.6	38	9.7	83
5.7	39	9.8	84
5.8	40	9.9	85
5.9	41	10.0	86
6.0	42	10.1	87
6.1	43	10.2	88
6.2	44	10.3	89
6.3	45	10.4	90
6.4	46	10.5	91
6.5	48	10.6	92
6.6	49	10.7	93
6.7	50	10.8	95
6.8	51	10.9	96
6.9	52	11.0	97
7.0	53	11.1	98
7.1	54	11.2	99
7.2	55	11.3	100
7.3	56	11.4	101
7.4	57	11.5	102
7.5	58	11.6	103
7.6	60	11.7	104
7.7	61	11.8	105
7.8	62	11.9	107
7.9	63	12.0	108
8.0	64		

NGSP, National Glycohemoglobin Standardization Program (United States); IFCC, International Federation of Clinical Chemistry.

MONITORING YOUR BLOOD SUGARS (mmol/L)

BASAL INSULIN

As you know, diabetes is a progressive disease and insulin needs can change. It is important to monitor for these changes so you can alter your insulin doses to keep your diabetes in good control.

Your basal insulin is _____

We recommend that:

1. You do not check your blood glucose every day.

2. However, for 1 week of every month check your blood glucose when you wake up.

    - If three or more of these seven blood glucose checks are

        < .... mmol/L, *decrease* your insulin dose by 10%.

    - If three or more of these seven blood glucose checks are

        > .... mmol/L, *increase* your insulin dose by 10%.

3. Two days before your scheduled diabetes check with your doctor:

    - Check your blood glucose before every meal and 2 hours after every meal.

    - Write these numbers down on paper, so that should your HbA_{1c} not be at target, your provider can review the sugars with you to work out what adjustments need to be made to your current management regime.

MONITORING YOUR BLOOD SUGARS (mg/dL)

BASAL INSULIN

As you know diabetes is a progressive disease and insulin needs can change.

It is important to monitor for these changes so you can alter your insulin doses to keep your diabetes in good control.

Your basal insulin is _____

We recommend that:

1. You do not check your blood glucose every day.

2. However, for 1 week of every month check your blood glucose when you wake up.

   - If three or more of these seven blood glucose checks are

     < .... mg/dL *decrease* your insulin dose by 10%.

   - If three or more of these three blood glucose checks are

     > .... mg/dL *increase* your insulin dose by 10%.

3. Two days before your scheduled diabetes check with your doctor:

   - Check your blood glucose before every meal and 2 hours after every meal.

   - Write these numbers down on paper, so that should your HbA_{1c} not be at target, your provider can review the sugars with you to work out what adjustments need to be made to your current management regime.

EXAMPLE OF A CORRECTION FACTOR (mmol/L)

Your correction factor: 1 unit of Humalog will lower your blood sugar by 1 mmol/L

Your goal blood sugar is 8 mmol/L

Your mealtime dose is 8 units

If your blood sugar is		Before meal (meal + correction)	After meal (correction only)
6	take	6 units	−2 units
7	take	7 units	−1 units
8	take	8 units	0 units
9	take	9 units	1 units
10	take	10 units	2 units
11	take	11 units	3 units
12	take	12 units	4 units
13	take	13 units	5 units
14	take	14 units	6 units
15	take	15 units	7 units
16	take	16 units	8 units
17	take	17 units	9 units
18	take	18 units	10 units
19	take	19 units	11 units
20	CALL	_____ (phone number)	

EXAMPLE OF A CORRECTION FACTOR (mg/dL)

Your correction factor: 1 unit of Humalog will lower your blood sugar by 20 mg/dL

Your goal blood sugar is 100 mg/dL

Your mealtime dose is 8 units

If your blood sugar is		Before meal (meal + correction)	After meal (correction only)
40	take	5 units	−3 units
60	take	6 units	−2 units
80	take	7 units	−1 units
100	take	8 units	0 units
120	take	9 units	1 units
140	take	10 units	2 units
160	take	11 units	3 units
180	take	12 units	4 units
200	take	13 units	5 units
220	take	14 units	6 units
240	take	15 units	7 units
260	take	16 units	8 units
280	take	17 units	9 units
300	take	18 units	10 units

300	CALL	_____
		(phone number)

FOODS

Carbohydrate	Protein	Fats	Fruit/vegetable

Flour
  Bread
  Scone
  Cake
  Biscuits
  Pastry
  Pasta
 	
Grains
  Rye, barley, wheat
  Quinoa
  Rice
  Breakfast cereals
 	
Sugar
  Chocolate/sweets
  Biscuits
  Jam
  Honey
  Juice/fizzy drinks
  Fruit
 	
Pulses
  Lentils
  Kidney beans
  Chickpeas
  Baked beans
 	
Potato
  Sweet potato
  Parsnip
  Pumpkin
  Taro
  Yams
 	
Some vegetables
  Corn
  Peas
	Meat
	  Pork
	  Lamb
	  Beef
	
	Poultry
	  Chicken
	  Turkey
	
	Fish
	  Tuna
	  Seafood
	
	Eggs
	  Mayonnaise
	
	Dairy
	  Yoghurt (plain)
	  Cheese
	  Cottage cheese
	  Cream cheese
	
	Soy
	  Tofu
	  Soya milk
	
	Nuts
	  Peanuts
	  Peanut butter
		Fat from meat
		  Lard
		  Dripping
		
		Oil
		  Fish oil
		  Olive oil
		  Corn oil
		  Coconut oil
		  Margarine
		  Salad dressing
		
		Dairy
		  Butter
		  Cream
		
		Avocado
			Leafy greens
			  Cabbage
			  Kale
			  Spinach
			  Spring greens
			  Swiss chard
			
			Green beans
			Carrots
			Broccoli
			Cauliflower
			
			Salad vegetables
			  Tomato
			  Lettuce
			  Cucumber
			  Radish
			  Pepper
			  Carrot

MANAGEMENT OF YOUR CARDIOVASCULAR RISK

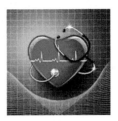

There are five important areas of health that we monitor and manage to ensure your heart and vascular system are being well looked after. Each of these can contribute to cardio-vascular disease, even more so in a patient with diabetes.

Where do you stand?

1. Diabetes
   Your HbA_{1c} target is _____ mmol/mol (%)   Yours_____

2. Smoking   Yes/No

3. High blood pressure
   BP < 140/90 mmHg   Yours_____

4. High cholesterol
   LDL (bad) < 1.8 mmol/L (70 mg/dL)   Yours_____

5. Obesity
   BMI (weight/height in m^2) < 25 kg/m^2 Yours_____

_____

We also want to make sure that your heart and kidneys are being protected.

Heart protection – aspirin/day   Yes/No
Kidney protection – ACE/ARB   Yes/No

WHAT IS A RETINAL SCREEN?

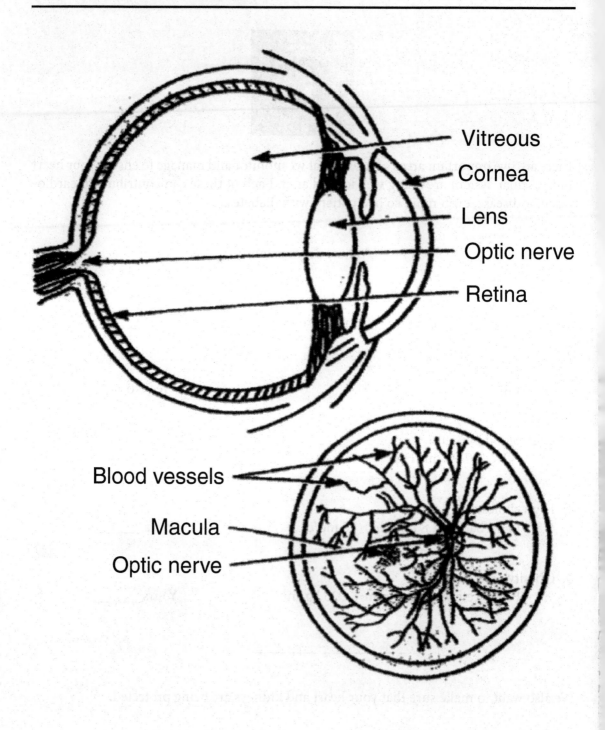

Vitreous

Cornea

Lens

Optic nerve

Retina

Blood vessels

Macula

Optic nerve